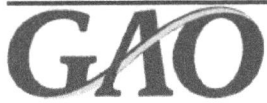

United States Government Accountability Office

Report to the Chairman, Committee on Environment and Public Works, U.S. Senate

August 2013

ENVIRONMENTAL HEALTH

EPA Has Made Substantial Progress but Could Improve Processes for Considering Children's Health

GAO-13-254

GAO Highlights

Highlights of GAO-13-254, a report to the Chairman, Committee on Environment and Public Works, U.S. Senate

ENVIRONMENTAL HEALTH

EPA Has Made Substantial Progress but Could Improve Processes for Considering Children's Health

Why GAO Did This Study

Scientific studies have shown that because children's bodies are still developing, they can be more vulnerable than adults to certain environmental hazards, including air pollutants, pesticide residues on food, contaminants in drinking water, and toxic chemicals in the home. EPA has made protecting children's health part of its mission by establishing a policy in 1995 to ensure that the agency consistently considers children in its actions and creating OCHP to support those efforts. In a 2010 report, GAO found that EPA had not fully utilized OCHP and other child-focused resources to protect children's health.

GAO was asked to review EPA's progress in protecting children's health. This report determines (1) the extent to which EPA has implemented GAO's 2010 recommendations on children's health protection and (2) the role, if any, that OCHP has played in ensuring that key EPA program offices consider children's health protection in their regulatory activities. The report also describes how OCHP has worked with external partners to leverage its resources. To conduct this work, GAO reviewed relevant laws and EPA regulations and guidance, analyzed EPA data, and interviewed EPA officials and other stakeholders.

What GAO Recommends

GAO recommends, among other things, that EPA direct OCHP and OPP to establish procedures to identify those tolerance decisions that could pose a significant risk to children's health and provide opportunities for OCHP involvement when appropriate. EPA generally agreed with GAO.

View GAO-13-254. For more information, contact David C. Trimble at (202) 512-3841 or trimbled@gao.gov.

What GAO Found

The Environmental Protection Agency (EPA) has made substantial progress in addressing more than half of the recommendations GAO made in a January 2010 report concerning the agency's efforts to protect children's health. Specifically, EPA has fully implemented five of the eight recommendations made by GAO. For example, for a recommendation that EPA ensure that its strategic plan expressly articulate children-specific goals, objectives, and targets, in September 2010, EPA issued an agency-wide strategic plan that identifies children's health as a top agency priority with goals, objectives, and targets. In addition, EPA took some steps to address the remaining three recommendations from GAO's January 2010 report but has not fully implemented them, including a recommendation that the agency strengthen the data system that identifies and tracks development of rulemakings and other actions to ensure they comply with the 1995 policy on evaluating health risks to children.

The Office of Children's Health Protection (OCHP) has increased its role to ensure that EPA program offices consider children's health protection in their regulatory activities. Specifically, the EPA Administrator issued a memorandum in February 2010 directing OCHP to take the lead in ensuring that all EPA programs are successful in their efforts to protect children's health. Since the issuance of the memorandum and the office's reorganization in July 2010, OCHP has played a greater supporting role in program offices' development of selected regulations that potentially affect children's health. However, OCHP has no regular involvement in the Office of Pesticide Program's (OPP) decision-making process addressing tolerances for pesticide residues. In addition, OCHP officials may not be aware of these decisions, and there are no mechanisms in the tolerance setting process to alert OCHP when matters that could pose a significant risk to children's health are being considered. Until the disconnect between the direction identified for OCHP in the Administrator's memorandum and the current process is addressed, OCHP will not have a role to ensure that children's health protection is considered in the area of pesticide tolerance decisions.

OCHP has worked extensively with a variety of partners to leverage its resources to better protect children's health. Through its coordination with federal partners, OCHP has helped to improve children's environmental health in schools and homes. For example, training courses for about 800 participants through the National Center for Healthy Housing are being offered around the country addressing topics such as pest management and energy efficiency. In addition, OCHP has financially supported children's health efforts in underserved communities across the country by providing grants totaling $1.2 million. For example, OCHP awarded a $100,000 grant to Farm Worker Justice, a group which provides outreach and educational activities for families of farm workers to improve the environmental health of their children. OCHP has also worked with Pediatric Environmental Health Specialty Units (PEHSU) to help train 15,000 health care providers across the country about the health implications of prenatal and childhood environmental exposures. PEHSUs also work with federal, state and local agencies to address children's environmental health issues in homes, schools, and communities.

Contents

Table

Figures

Abbreviations

ADP	Action Development Process
CBI	confidential business information
CDC	Centers for Disease Control and Prevention
CHPAC	Children's Health Protection Advisory Committee
DFO	Designated Federal Officer
EPA	Environmental Protection Agency
FACA	Federal Advisory Committee Act
Forum	Federal Interagency Forum on Child and Family Statistics
FQPA	Food Quality Protection Act of 1996
FTE	full-time equivalent
HHS	Department of Health and Human Services
IG	Inspector General
LOAEL	Lowest observed adverse effect level
National Agenda	National Agenda to Protect Children's Health from Environmental Threats
NRDC	Natural Resources Defense Council
OCHP	Office of Children's Health Protection
OPP	Office of Pesticide Programs
PEHSU	Pediatric Environmental Health Specialty Unit
SDWA	Safe Drinking Water Act Amendments of 1996

August 12, 2013

The Honorable Barbara Boxer
Chairman
Committee on Environment and Public Works
United States Senate

Dear Madam Chairman:

Scientific studies have shown that because children's bodies are still developing, they can be more vulnerable than adults to certain environmental hazards, including air pollutants, pesticide residues on food, contaminants in drinking water, and toxic chemicals found in the home.[1] Children's vulnerability to environmental hazards may also stem from their behavior, which can expose them to such hazards. For example, air pollutants such as ozone that may produce serious complications in children and adults with lung diseases, including asthma, may be more likely to affect children, in part because their airways and lungs are still developing and they spend more time outdoors.[2] Additionally, children's exposure to some chemical hazards may be greater than adults' because infants and young children engage in more hand-to-mouth behavior, and spend more time on the floor, where some of these hazards (e.g., lead dust) are more likely to be.[3] According to a

---

[1] M. Herrmann, K. King, and M. Weitzman. "Prenatal Tobacco Smoke and Postnatal Secondhand Smoke Exposure and Child Neurodevelopment," *Current Opinion in Pediatrics* 20, no. 2 (2008):184-190. B. Weiss and D.C. Bellinger, "Social Ecology of Children's Vulnerability to Environmental Pollutants," *Environmental Health Perspectives* 114, no. 10 (2006): 1,479-1,485.

[2] Approximately 7 million children in the United States have asthma, according to the President's Task Force on Environmental Health Risks and Safety Risks to Children, and asthma accounted for 10.5 million missed school days in 2008. L.J. Akinbami, J.E. Mooreman, C. Bailey, H. Zahran, M. King, C. Johnson, & X. Liu. Centers for Disease Control and Prevention, National Center for Health Statistics (2012). "Trends in Asthma Prevalence, Health Care Use, and Mortality in the United States, 2001-2010." Retrieved from http://www.cdc. gov/nchs/data/databriefs/db94.pdf.

[3] Children are particularly susceptible to accidental poisoning because they tend to play on floors and explore by putting items in their mouths. EPA takes action to address such hazards. For example, in February 2013, EPA initiated a regulatory action to cancel and remove from the consumer market 12 D-Con brand mouse and rat poison bait products. At the manufacturer's request, EPA will hold a pesticide cancellation hearing which will determine whether a final cancellation notice will be issued. Documentation is available in docket EPA-HQ-OPP-2013-0049 at www.regulations.gov.

January 2012 report from the Department of Health and Human Service's Centers for Disease Control and Prevention (CDC),[4] approximately 450,000 children in the United States have elevated levels of lead in their blood, and lead exposure may cause learning disabilities or health problems in their cardiovascular, immunological, and endocrine systems.[5] Relative to their body weight, children also breathe more air, drink more water, and consume more food than adults. Ongoing research continues to increase our understanding of children's vulnerabilities. Studies have also shown that early life exposures to environmental hazards may increase risk of some diseases later on in life. For example, several studies have reported associations between exposure to harmful contaminants in early life and adverse health effects such as neurodevelopmental disorders.[6] According to the Environmental Protection Agency's (EPA) January 2013 *America's Children and Environment* report, childhood leukemia, in particular, has been associated with exposures to pesticides.[7] In addition, the report states that childhood exposures to certain pesticides have been associated with neurodevelopmental effects such as attention-deficit/hyperactivity disorder and learning disabilities.

EPA has promoted children's environmental health protection in an increasing number of ways over the past three decades. According to EPA officials, since the 1970s its national ambient air quality reviews have integrated protection of children and other at-risk populations. For example, in 1978 EPA set a National Ambient Air Quality Standard for

---

[4]CDC, Advisory Committee on Childhood Lead Poisoning Prevention Report, January 4, 2012.

[5]Although no "safe" threshold of exposure has ever been identified, levels above 5 micrograms per deciliter of blood (μg/dL) are considered elevated, according to the CDC.

[6] Y. Lambrinidou, S. Triantafyllidou, and M. Edwards, "Failing our Children: Lead in U.S. School Drinking Water,"*New Solutions: A Journal of Environmental and Occupational Health Policy* 20, no. 1 (2010): 25-47; D.E. Jacobs, R.P. Clickner, J.Y. Zhou, S.M. Viet, D.A. Marker, J.W. Rogers, D.C. Zeldin, P. Broene, and W. Friedman, "The Prevalence of Lead-Based Paint Hazards in U.S. Housing," *Environmental Health Perspectives* 110, no. 10 (2002): A599-606; N. Ribas-Fito, M. Sala, M. Kogevinas, and J. Sunyer, "Polychlorinated Biphenyls (PCBs) and Neurological Development in Children: a Systematic Review,"*Journal of Epidemiology and Community Health* 55, no. 8 (2001): 537-546.

[7]EPA, *America's Children and the Environment*, 3rd ed. (Washington, D.C.: January 2013).

GAO-13-254 EPA Children's Health

lead based on particular concerns about children's sensitivity.[8] In 1995, in response to new data regarding the potential adverse effects of environmental hazards on children, EPA established an agency-wide policy to ensure that the agency consistently and explicitly considers children in developing risk assessments, and environmental and public health standards. In 1997, EPA created the Office of Children's Health Protection (OCHP) to support the agency's efforts and formed the Children's Health Protection Advisory Committee (CHPAC) to provide advice, information, and recommendations to assist the agency in developing regulations, guidance, and policies relevant to children's health.

In roughly the same time frame as the creation of OCHP, two key legislative requirements were enacted and an executive order was signed to further protect children's health. Both the Safe Drinking Water Act Amendments of 1996 (SDWA) and the Food Quality Protection Act of 1996 (FQPA) were enacted with explicit provisions for considering children's health in the decision-making process for certain regulatory actions. SDWA, as amended, requires that EPA, in selecting a maximum contaminant level (i.e., an enforceable limit for a contaminant in drinking water), must analyze the effects on vulnerable groups, such as infants, children, pregnant women, the elderly, individuals with a history of serious illness, or other subpopulations that are identified as likely to be at greater risk.[9] Similarly, in selecting contaminants to consider for regulation, SDWA requires EPA to consider the effects on vulnerable subgroups, such as infants, children, and pregnant women that comprise a meaningful portion of the general population but are at higher risk.[10] FQPA provides heightened protections for infants and children, directing EPA, in setting pesticide tolerances (i.e., the maximum legal amount of a pesticide residue that is allowed to remain on a food commodity that has been treated with the pesticide), to use an additional default 10-fold margin of safety to protect infants and children—unless data support a

---

[8]EPA has set National Ambient Air Quality Standards for six pollutants, termed "criteria" pollutants: carbon monoxide, lead, nitrogen oxide, ozone, particulate matter, and sulfur dioxides.

[9]42 U.S.C. § 300g-1(b)(3)(C)(i)(V)(2013).

[10]42 U.S.C. § 300g-1(b)(1)(C)(2013).

different margin—taking into account the potential for pre- and postnatal toxicity and other factors.[11]

About a decade later, additional legislation was enacted relevant to EPA activities to protect children's environmental health in schools. The Energy Independence and Security Act of 2007 requires that EPA—in consultation with the Department of Education, the Department of Health and Human Services (HHS)[12] and other relevant agencies—develop voluntary guidelines to assist states in establishing and implementing environmental health programs in schools. The Energy Independence and Security Act also requires that EPA develop, in consultation with the Department of Education and HHS, voluntary guidelines for locating schools that are, among other things, to take into account the special vulnerability of children to environmental hazards.

We and EPA's Office of Inspector General have raised concerns about the effectiveness of EPA's actions to protect children's health. In a January 2010 report, we found that EPA had not fully utilized OCHP and other child-focused resources and that it did not have a high-level strategy or dedicated resources for outreach and coordination.[13] More generally, we found that EPA needed a high-level strategy for children's health and greater leadership to make continued progress in protecting children from environmental threats. We recommended that the agency update and reissue a child-focused strategy, reevaluate the mission of OCHP and its Director, and take other steps to help ensure that EPA assumes high-level leadership and develops strategies and structures for coordinating efforts addressing children's environmental health. EPA concurred with our recommendations and agreed to implement them. An

---

[11]21 U.S.C. §346a(b)(2)(A)(standard for pesticides residues with a threshold effect), (b)(2)(C)(exposure of infants and children), (c)(2) (exemptions).

[12]In particular, within HHS, the Agency for Toxic Substances and Disease Registry is respons ble for investigating community exposures related to certain hazardous chemical sites and releases; assessing associated health effects; recommending actions to stop, prevent, or minimize harmful effects; and conducting health studies.

[13]GAO, *Environmental Health:* High-level Strategy and Leadership Needed to Continue Progress toward Protecting Children from Environmental Threats, GAO-10-205 (Washington, D.C.: Jan. 28, 2010). In an earlier report, we recommended that EPA proactively use its children's health advisory committee; see GAO, Environmental Health: *EPA Efforts to Address Children's Health Issues Need Greater Focus, Direction, and Top-level Commitment*, GAO-08-1155T (Washington, D.C.: Sept. 16, 2008).

EPA Inspector General (IG) report issued that same year made similar recommendations.[14]

In February 2010, EPA's Administrator issued a memorandum reaffirming that the agency's policy is to consider the health of pregnant women, infants, and children consistently and explicitly in all activities related to human-health protection, including performing risk assessments and setting standard practices. The Administrator also directed OCHP to take the lead in ensuring that EPA programs and regions are successful in their efforts to protect children's health. OCHP's current strategic plan reiterates that the office's mission will be accomplished by providing leadership in identifying critical agency actions to protect children's environmental health, among other efforts.

In light of these developments, you asked us to examine EPA's progress in protecting children's health. Specifically, this report determines (1) the extent to which EPA has implemented our 2010 recommendations concerning children's health protection and (2) the role, if any, that OCHP has played in ensuring that key EPA program offices consider children's health protection in their regulatory activities. The report also describes how OCHP has worked with external partners to leverage its resources to better protect children's health.

To conduct this work, we reviewed relevant laws, regulations, and EPA guidance and interviewed senior officials at EPA headquarters. We also interviewed other stakeholders, including members of CHPAC and representatives of various children's health advocacy groups, including the National Center for Healthy Housing; Healthy Schools Network, Inc.; and the National Environmental Education Foundation. More specifically, to determine the extent that EPA has addressed our 2010 recommendations concerning children's health, we interviewed key officials from OCHP and EPA's Office of Policy, as well as members of CHPAC. Additionally, we attended two CHPAC meetings held in November 2011 and March 2012. We also reviewed EPA's fiscal years 2011-2015 strategic plan and other planning and guidance documents. To better understand OCHP's role and responsibilities in ensuring that key program offices consider children's health protection in their

---

[14]EPA Office of the Inspector General, *Need Continues for a Strategic Plan to Protect Children's Health*, 10-P-0095 (Washington, D.C.: Apr. 5, 2010).

regulatory activities, we relied on OCHP's analysis from fiscal year 2011 based on the measures included in its fiscal years 2011-2013 strategic plan.[15] We also interviewed workgroup participants on selected regulations analyzed by OCHP, including EPA program offices with lead responsibility for selected actions. Moreover, we interviewed key program officials at EPA that have statutory responsibility for addressing children's health. Specifically, we interviewed officials from EPA's Office of Water and Office of Pesticide Programs (OPP) to assess their efforts to protect children's health under SDWA and FQPA, respectively. Additionally, to assess the reliability of summary data on OPP's decisions to retain or alter the default 10-fold margin of safety from 1996 to 2012 that OPP provided to us, we interviewed OPP officials who maintain the data on pesticide tolerances, among other things, and determined that the data were sufficiently reliable for the purposes of this report. We also interviewed environmental health experts to get additional perspective on EPA's children's health efforts. To determine how OCHP has worked with external partners to leverage its resources to better protect children's health, we reviewed and analyzed key EPA documents involving outreach and coordination. We focused on OCHP's efforts to work with community-based programs, train health care providers, and conduct research. We also reviewed budget documents and interviewed EPA officials and members of external organizations about OCHP's outreach and coordination efforts. For more detail on our objectives, scope, and methodology, see appendix I.

We conducted this performance audit from November 2011 to August 2013 in accordance with generally accepted government auditing standards. Those standards require that we plan and perform the audit to obtain sufficient, appropriate evidence to provide a reasonable basis for our findings and conclusions based on our audit objectives. We believe that the evidence obtained provides a reasonable basis for our findings and conclusions based on our audit objectives.

Background

EPA's mission is to protect human health and the environment. The agency ensures that all Americans are protected from significant risks to human health and the environment where they live, work and play. As

---

[15]This was the most recent period for which information was available when we began our work.

part of its mission, EPA states that protecting children's health from environmental risks is fundamental to EPA's mission and that the agency reduces negative environmental impacts on children through involvement in EPA rulemakings, policy, enforcement actions, research, and applications of science that focus on prenatal and childhood vulnerabilities. EPA views childhood as a sequence of life stages from conception through maternal/fetal development, infancy, and adolescence. These lifestages refer to a distinguishable time frame in an individual's life characterized by unique and relatively stable behavioral or physiological characteristics that are associated with development and growth.[16]

EPA's Early Actions to Address Children's Environmental Health

In 1995, EPA established an agency-wide Policy on Evaluating Health Risks to Children, directing EPA staff to consistently and explicitly consider risks to infants and children as a part of risk assessments generated during its decision-making processes, and when setting standards to protect public health and the environment (see app. II). In 1996, EPA issued the National Agenda to Protect Children's Health from Environmental Threats (National Agenda) and expanded the agency's activities to specifically address risks for children.

In 1997, EPA established OCHP, within the Office of the Administrator, to support and facilitate the agency's efforts to implement its National Agenda. OCHP's mission was originally to make the protection of children's health a fundamental goal of public health and environmental protection in the United States and around the world. Since this time, the office's mission has become more focused. According to OCHP's 2010 strategic plan, the office's current mission is to "ensure EPA actions and programs further the protection of children's environmental health," and this mission is supported with the following four goals:

- Goal 1: Reduce negative environmental health impacts on children through rulemaking, policy, enforcement actions, research, and application of science that focuses on prenatal and childhood vulnerabilities.

---

[16]EPA, *Guidance on Selecting Age Groups for Monitoring and Assessing Childhood Exposures to Environmental Contaminants*, EPA/630/P-03003F (Washington, D.C.: November 2005).

- Goal 2: Protect children through safe chemicals management.

- Goal 3: Coordinate national and international community-based programs to eliminate threats to children's health.

- Goal 4: Measure and communicate progress on children's environmental health.

Based on EPA's fiscal year 2012 enacted budget, to accomplish its mission and goals, OCHP has staff resources of 18.2 full-time equivalents (FTE) in headquarters and the regions, including the Director, and a budget of approximately $7.48 million.[17] To inform its various initiatives related to children's health, EPA also established CHPAC in 1997. Through CHPAC, leading researchers, academics, health care providers, nongovernmental organizations, industry representatives, as well as state and local government representatives, advise EPA on regulations, research, and communication issues important to children's health.

| Executive Order 13045— Protection of Children from Environmental Health Risks and Safety Risks | The President issued an executive order in April 1997 that established a broad policy for a concerted federal effort to address children's environmental health risks and safety risks.[18] The executive order required each federal agency to (1) make it a high priority to identify and assess environmental health risks and safety risks that may disproportionately affect children and (2) ensure that its policies, programs, activities, and standards address disproportionate risks to children that result from environmental health risks or safety risks. The executive order requires federal agencies to develop two pieces of information as part of the rulemaking process: (1) an evaluation of the environmental health or safety effects on children of the planned rule and (2) an explanation of why the planned rule is preferable to other potentially effective and reasonably feasible alternatives considered by the agency. The requirements of the executive order are triggered if a rulemaking is likely to result in a rule that (1) may be economically significant, such as by having an annual impact on the economy of $100 |

---

[17]An FTE generally consists of one or more employees who collectively complete 2,080 work hours in a given year. Therefore, either one full-time employee or two half-time employees equal one FTE.

[18]Executive Order 13045 § 2-202 (a) -(b), 62 Fed. Reg. 19,885 (Apr. 23, 1997).

GAO-13-254 EPA Children's Health

million or more, and (2) concerns an environmental health risk or safety risk that an agency has reason to believe may disproportionately affect children.

Statutory Requirements to Consider Children's Environmental Health

In addition to the broad mandate to protect children's health that was established by the President in Executive Order 13045, EPA is specifically directed by Congress to consider infants and children in two environmental statutes—SDWA, as amended, and FQPA.[19]

The Safe Drinking Water Act

Overview of requirements: Under SDWA,[20] as amended, EPA is authorized to regulate contaminants in public drinking water systems. The act requires that EPA identify and publish a list every 5 years of unregulated contaminants that may require regulation, called the contaminant candidate list. For at least five contaminants every 5 years, EPA is then to evaluate their occurrence, and the potential health risks associated with them, and decide whether a regulation is needed; these decisions on whether to regulate a contaminant are known as regulatory determinations. In listing contaminants and in considering them for regulatory determination, EPA is to select contaminants that present "the greatest public health concern," taking into consideration effects on sensitive populations—such as children—that are identifiable as at greater risk of adverse health effects from exposure to contaminants in drinking water, among other factors. [21]

Establishing drinking water standards: For contaminants that EPA has determined to regulate or been directed to regulate, EPA establishes legally enforceable standards for public water systems—called national primary drinking water regulations—which generally limit the levels of specific contaminants in drinking water that can adversely affect public health. In proposing such standards, SDWA requires EPA to prepare and use, among other things, an analysis of the effects of the contaminant at

---

[19]EPA considers children in undertaking actions under a broad range of statutes; in some instances, other statutes do not explicitly require consideration of impacts of the action on children, but their legislative histories may do so. For example, the Clean Air Act does not explicitly require special consideration of susceptible subgroups when setting the National Ambient Air Quality Standards, but its legislative history indicates the standard is to be set to protect the health of any sensitive group of the population.

[20]Pub. L. No. 93-523, 88 Stat. 1660 (1974) (codified as amended at 42 U.S.C. §§ 300f–300j-26). Hereinafter, references to SDWA sections are as amended.

[21]42 U.S.C. § 300g-1(b)(1)(C) (2013).

sensitive life stages—such as for infants, children, and pregnant women—that may have a greater risk of adverse health effects from exposure to the contaminants in drinking water than the general population.[22] EPA's Office of Water has primary responsibility for implementing these requirements of SDWA.

The Food Quality Protection Act

Overview of requirements: FQPA amended section 408 of the Federal Food, Drug and Cosmetic Act (FFDCA), by adding several new requirements including a new safety standard for establishing levels of pesticide residue on raw and processed food. Under FFDCA, a pesticide[23] chemical residue is deemed unsafe in or on food unless EPA has established either a tolerance (i.e., the maximum legal amount of a pesticide residue that is allowed to remain on a food commodity that has been treated with the pesticide) or exemption from the requirement for a tolerance and the level of residues is within the tolerance or exemption.[24] Since FQPA was enacted in 1996, EPA may establish a tolerance only if the Administrator determines that the tolerance is safe (i.e., that there is a reasonable certainty that no harm will result from exposure to the pesticide residue from all food and nonfood sources).[25] EPA may establish, amend, or revoke a tolerance for a pesticide; we refer to these collectively as tolerance decisions. These tolerance decisions may be made in conjunction with pesticide registrations, registration review, or

---

[22] 42 U.S.C. § 300g-1(b)(3)(C)(i)(V) (2013).

[23] A pesticide is a substance intended to repel, kill, or control any species designated a "pest" including weeds, insects, rodents, fungi, bacteria, or other organisms. The family of pesticides includes herbicides, insecticides, rodenticides, fungicides, and bactericides. A pesticide residue is a residue of pesticide left in or on food after application of the pesticide.

[24] 21 U.S.C. § 346a(a)(1) (2013). In this report, references to FFDCA are generally to section 408.

[25] 21 U.S.C. § 346a(b)(2)(A) (2013). Specifically, a tolerance is "safe" if the Administrator has determined that there is a reasonable certainty that no harm will result from aggregate exposure to the pesticide chemical residue, including all anticipated dietary exposures and all other exposures for which there is reliable information. Similarly, EPA may establish an exemption from the requirement for a tolerance only if the Administrator determines that the exemption is safe; the term 'safe' means that the Administrator has determined that there is a reasonable certainty that no harm will result from aggregate exposure to the pesticide chemical residue, including all anticipated dietary exposures and all other exposures for which there is reliable information. *Id.* at (c)(2)(A).

reregistrations.[26] These tolerance decisions may be initiated by submissions, called petitions, received from industry or the public; or independently by EPA. These actions are taken pursuant to section 408 of FFDCA, which governs pesticide residues on food, among other things, and the Federal Insecticide, Fungicide, and Rodenticide Act that governs pesticide registration. For example, EPA may establish a tolerance as part of a new use registration, such as when a pesticide manufacturer seeks approval for use of an existing pesticide on a different food crop. Similarly, EPA may amend a tolerance when a pesticide manufacturer completes studies that were not available at the time the existing tolerance was set. According to EPA officials, generally, in both of these instances, the tolerance process would be initiated by a petition from the pesticide registrant.

Establishing pesticide tolerances: In establishing or reviewing a tolerance, OPP is to combine information on pesticide toxicity (i.e., the degree to which a pesticide is harmful or deadly) with information regarding the route, magnitude, frequency, and duration of exposure to the pesticide through a risk assessment process. The risk assessment process involves the following four distinct steps:

- identification of the toxicological hazards posed by a pesticide;

- determination of the "level of concern" with respect to human exposure to the pesticide, including determination and application of safety factors;

- estimation of human exposure to the pesticide; and

- characterization of risk posed to humans by the pesticide based on comparison of human exposure to the level of concern.

---

[26] Under the Federal Insecticide, Fungicide, and Rodenticide Act, as amended, EPA registers pesticides for distribution, sale, and use in the United States and prescribes labeling and other regulatory requirements to prevent unreasonable adverse effects on the environment. To obtain a registration, a company or person (registrant) must submit health and environmental effects data and other information for EPA's review. If the registration is for a food use pesticide, the applicant must also submit a petition for all needed tolerances. EPA may register the pesticide and set a tolerance level for those pesticides used on food or animal feed, notify the registrant of deficiencies in the data or need for additional information, or reject the application.

Thus, at the conclusion of the risk assessment process, OPP will establish a tolerance only if estimated exposure under the tolerance is below the level of concern. As amended by FQPA, FFDCA mandates that, in taking action on a tolerance, EPA assess risks to infants and children from the pesticide chemical residue, among other things. Specifically, FFDCA requires that, in taking actions on tolerances, including exemptions, EPA is to assess the risk of the pesticide chemical residue based on available information about consumption patterns among infants and children where disproportionate; the special susceptibility of infants and children to the residues; and the cumulative effects on infants and children of such residues and other substances that have a common mechanism of toxicity. Further EPA is to ensure that "there is a reasonable certainty that no harm will result to infants and children from aggregate exposure to the pesticide chemical residue" and publish a specific determination regarding the safety of the pesticide chemical residue for infants and children.[27]

Applying an FQPA safety factor. FFDCA requires that when setting a tolerance that EPA apply "an additional default 10-fold margin of safety for the pesticide chemical residue and other sources of exposure . . . for infants and children to take into account potential pre- and post-natal toxicity and completeness of the data with respect to exposure and toxicity to infants and children."[28] The statute provides the Administrator with the authority to apply a different margin of safety for a pesticide chemical residue if, on the basis of reliable data, such a margin would be safe for infants and children.[29] In other words, EPA can only apply a safety factor other than the default 10-fold if data demonstrate that such a margin will be safe. Because this requirement of an additional safety factor was added to FFDCA by FQPA, it is commonly referred to as the FQPA safety factor. OPP interpreted these 1996 FPQA provisions in key

---

[27]Pub. L. No. 104-170 § 405, 110 Stat. 1514 (Aug. 3, 1996) (amending FFDCA §408, 21 U.S.C. § 346a) (codified at 21 U.S.C. § 346a(b)(2)(C)).

[28]Id. This provision is applicable to pesticides with threshold effects.

[29]Id.

2002 guidance.[30] According to OPP's 2002 guidance, the FQPA default 10-fold children's safety factor provision "both codifies and expands OPP's past practice of applying uncertainty factors to account for deficiencies in the toxicological database."[31] The guidance also explains how OPP will approach analyzing the body of data on a particular pesticide to determine whether to apply the default 10-fold safety factor to protect infants and children or to apply another safety factor. Per the guidance, OPP's approach to this analysis is to consist of several key considerations as follows:

1. Completeness of the toxicity database—whether all the required toxicity studies on the pesticide have been submitted.

2. Completeness of the exposure database—whether the exposure data on the pesticide are complete.

3. Potential pre- and postnatal sensitivity—whether fetuses and infants may be particularly sensitive to health effects of the pesticide. For example, EPA may use results of reproductive or developmental studies to determine this sensitivity or other evidence regarding whether fetuses or children would tend to be more susceptible considering the nature of the pesticide's health effects.

Presumption to apply safety factor. In its guidance, OPP states that the office is to interpret these statutory directives as essentially establishing a presumption in favor of applying an additional default 10-fold safety factor to pesticide risk assessments. However, the guidance also notes that it is just a presumption. According to the guidance, OPP is to consider the available data and determine whether there is reliable evidence demonstrating that a different safety factor is protective. Moreover, FQPA requires the agency to publish its determination that a pesticide chemical residue is safe for infants and children. According to OPP officials, OPP's rationale for a tolerance decision is generally presented in EPA's *Federal Register* notices for the proposed or final tolerance decision.

---

[30]EPA, Office of Pesticide Programs, "Determination of the Appropriate FQPA Safety Factor(s) in Tolerance Assessment" (2002). In 2003, OPP supplemented the 2002 guidance in "Clarification on the Application of Database Uncertainty Factors as Described in the 2002 OPP FQPA 10X Guidance." In 2008, OPP's Health Effects Division, supplemented the 2002 guidance further with "Hot Sheet 30" ("Application of the FQPA safety factor in FFDCA risk assessments and additional uncertainty factors in FIFRA risk assessments").

[31]Id.

Reassessing existing pesticide tolerances: When the law was enacted in 1996, FQPA also required EPA to reassess, using the new safety standard, the more than 9,700 existing tolerances for pesticide residues on foods for the pesticides that were already registered. According to EPA officials, the agency completed the reassessments required by FQPA.[32]

Internal review of safety factors: OPP's decisions regarding whether to reduce, retain, or increase the FQPA safety factor for a specific pesticide are reviewed internally by the office's Toxicology Science Advisory Council, and its internal Risk Assessment Review Committee is responsible for validating these decisions.

EPA Action Development Process

EPA develops rules, regulations, and other agency actions through its Action Development Process (ADP).[33] The ADP is a defined and well-established agency process for developing rules that provide for interagency involvement through participation in regulatory workgroups to ensure that scientific, economic, and policy issues are adequately addressed at appropriate stages. At specific points in rule development, the ADP provides opportunities for senior management to get involved early and to provide guidance and direction to staff. EPA finalized the current process in June 2004 and updated its guidance in March 2011.[34] The overall process includes the following key activities:

- EPA assigns each action to one of three tiers based on the required level of cross-agency interaction, which is determined by reviewing the complexity, environmental and economic significance, and likely

[32]Currently there are more than 1,055 active ingredients registered as pesticides, which are formulated into thousands of pesticide products that are available in the marketplace, according to an EPA website.

[33]Office of Policy officials told us that the ADP generally applies to actions that are signed by the Administrator and/or appear in the Regulatory Agenda. These officials also noted that pesticide tolerance decisions are not signed by the Administrator and for the past two decades have not appeared in EPA's semiannual regulatory agenda, which states that it excludes routine actions such as pesticide tolerance decisions. EPA stated that for these reasons, pesticide tolerance decisions do not follow the ADP.

[34]*EPA's Action Development Process: Guidance for EPA Staff on Developing Quality Actions*, revised March 2011.

external interest in the action;[35] for example, EPA assigns actions that are based on a human risk assessment—including assessments of environmental health risks to children—to tier 1 or tier 2.

- The lead program office for an action follows a standard process to develop the proposed regulation and supporting analyses. For example, the lead program office convenes the workgroup that develops and drafts the action through such key tasks as (1) creating the analytical blueprint that spells out a workgroup's plans for the data collection and analyses that will support development of a specific action, (2) completing data gathering, and (3) developing and presenting options that best achieve the goal of the action.

In October 2006, the Office of Policy issued additional guidance developed by OCHP to assist agency staff in integrating children's health considerations into the rulemaking process.[36] The children's guidance describes provisions of Executive Order 13045 and EPA's Policy on Evaluating Health Risks to Children. Figure 1 illustrates key steps in EPA's ADP where children are to be considered by the agency.

---

[35]Tier 1 includes top actions that demand the ongoing involvement of the Administrator's office and extensive cross-agency involvement. Tier 2 actions include significant science, policy, economic or other implementation issues where primary decision authority rests with lead program or regional offices. Tier 3 actions are those for which little cross-agency participation is needed and lead offices can design their own review processes.

[36]*EPA's Action Development Process Guide to Considering Children's Health When Developing EPA Actions: Implementing Executive Order 13045 and EPA's Policy on Evaluating Health Risks to Children*, March 2006.

Figure 1: Steps Where Children Are Considered in the EPA Rulemaking Process

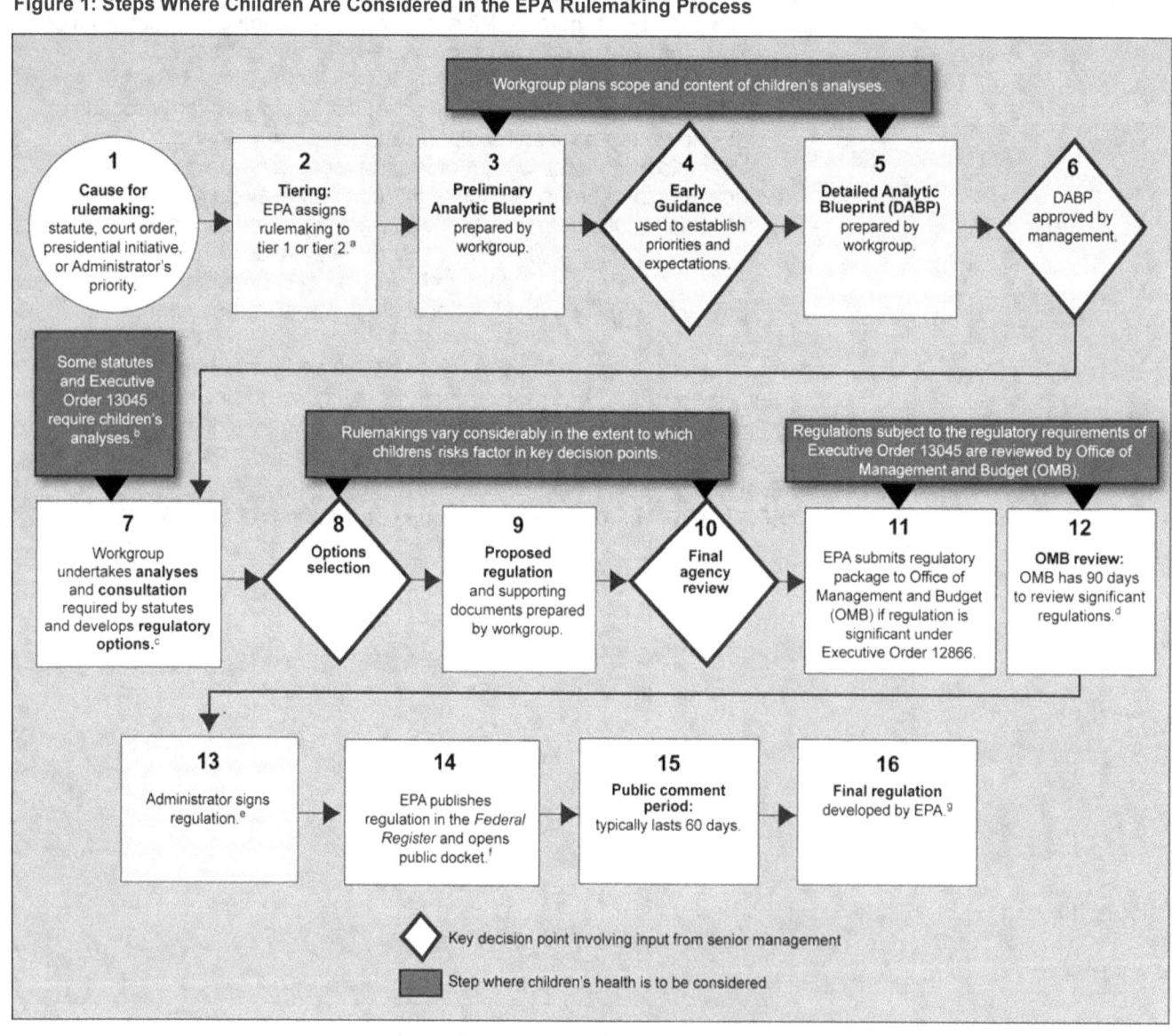

Source: GAO analysis of EPA's Action Development Process.

Note: In 1997, the President signed Executive Order (E.O.) 13045—Protection of Children from Environmental Health Risks and Safety Risks, which mandated a concerted federal effort to address children's environmental health and safety risks. Early Guidance from EPA management is used to establish policy priorities and communicate expectations for the workgroup. A Preliminary Analytic Blueprint is a document that spells out a workgroup's plans for the data collection and analyses that will support development of a specific action. The Detailed Analytic Blueprint is based on the Preliminary Analytic Blueprint. It is modified as necessary as a result of early guidance and should identify the key activities, analyses, consultation activities, contributors, and timelines.

^aThe children's health questions are addressed during the tiering process, step 2.

^bBoth the Safe Drinking Water Act, as amended, and the Federal Food, Drug, and Cosmetic Act, as amended by the Food Quality Protection Act, include specific provisions requiring EPA to consider infants and children.

^cThe 1995 Children's Health Policy is considered during workgroup analysis and consultation, step 7.

^dEPA may request a one-time 30-day extension.

^eThe Administrator may delegate signature authority to an Assistant or Associate Administrator or Regional Administrator.

^fA docket can be established at any time during the rulemaking process, but it should open no later than the date of publication in the *Federal Register*. A docket should contain all information relied upon by EPA in developing an action.

^gDeveloping the final regulation involves reconvening the workgroup to evaluate comments received on the proposal and determine the appropriate next steps for preparing the final action, which could range from repeating all of the steps as outlined in the process for preparing the proposal to only doing a subset of those steps.

EPA Has Made Substantial Progress in Addressing More than Half of Our 2010 Recommendations

EPA has made substantial progress in addressing our 2010 recommendations concerning the agency's efforts to protect children's health but has not fully implemented some of them. As figure 2 indicates, EPA has fully implemented five of the eight recommendations we made in January 2010 and has taken steps to address the remaining three recommendations.[37]

---

[37]GAO-10-205.

Figure 2: Implementation Status of GAO's 2010 Recommendations

Status	Recommendation
●	**Update and reissue a child-focused strategy**—such as the 1996 National Agenda, to articulate current national environmental health priorities and emerging issues.
●	**Ensure EPA's current strategic plan expressly articulates children-specific goals, objectives, and targets.**
●	**Reevaluate the mission of Office of Children's Health Protection (OCHP) and its Director.**
●	**Use the Children's Health Protection Advisory Committee proactively** as a mechanism for providing advice on regulations, programs, plans, or other issues.
●	**Ensure participation**—to the fullest extent possible, by Office of Children's Health Protection (OCHP) or other key officials **on the interagency organizations mentioned in Executive Order 13045.**
◐	**Strengthen the data system**—that identifies and tracks development of rulemakings and other actions to ensure they comply with the 1995 policy on children's health.
◐	**Reevaluate the 1995 policy**—to ensure its consistency with new scientific research demonstrating the risks childhood exposures can pose for disease in later lifestages.
◐	**Establish key children's environmental health staff within each program and regional office**—with linkages to Office of Children's Health Protection (OCHP) to improve cross-agency implementation of revised priorities and goals, and ensure coordination.

● Recommendation has been fully implemented

◐ Steps have been taken to implement recommendation, but recommendation has not been fully implemented

Source: GAO analysis of EPA information.

EPA Has Fully Implemented Five GAO Recommendations on Children's Health Protection

EPA has fully implemented five of our eight 2010 recommendations by taking the following actions:

EPA Issued a Children's Health Agenda Reflecting National Environmental Priorities and Emerging Issues

In our January 2010 report,[38] we recommended that the EPA Administrator update and reissue a child-focused strategy that would articulate current national health priorities and emerging issues. To address our recommendation, the EPA Administrator issued a memorandum in February 2010 that reaffirmed the agency's commitment to children's health and also detailed a three-point EPA Children's Health Agenda designed to, among other things, help ensure that EPA's actions address the environmental origins of health problems in children. A copy of the 2010 memorandum is provided in appendix III. Specifically, the memorandum states that "it is EPA's policy to consider the health of pregnant women, infants and children consistently and explicitly in all activities we undertake related to human-health protection, both domestically and internationally." The following are descriptions of EPA's February 2010 Children's Health Agenda (in the memorandum), which outlines three priorities for the agency:

- *Use the best science when developing regulations.* EPA will use the best science in efforts to implement the nation's environmental laws. EPA will robustly and transparently address the potential for and uniqueness of health effects in children when developing regulations and agency policies with human health implications. EPA will work with states and tribes to ensure that regulations are effectively implemented and enforced and will work closely with external research partners to fill critical data gaps.

- *Protect children through safe chemicals management.* EPA will protect children through safe chemicals management. EPA will establish standards, policies, and guidance at home and abroad that help eliminate harmful prenatal and childhood exposures to pesticides and other toxic chemicals and work with Congress and stakeholders to identify effective approaches for the protection of children's health in the context of the Toxic Substances Control Act (TSCA) reform.[39]

- *Coordinate national and international community-based programs to eliminate threats to children's health.* EPA will coordinate national and international community-based programs to eliminate threats to

---

[38]GAO-10-205.

[39]In 1976, Congress passed TSCA to provide EPA with the authority to obtain more information on chemicals and to regulate those chemicals that EPA determines pose unreasonable risks to human health or the environment.

children's health and measure and communicate progress; EPA will expand implementation of successful community-based programs to protect and improve children's health outcomes and will focus on underserved communities.

EPA Issued a Strategic Plan Incorporating Children's Health Protection

In our January 2010 report, we recommended that EPA ensure that its current strategic plan expressly articulates children-specific goals, objectives, and targets.[40] EPA's agency-wide strategic plan for fiscal years 2011-2015, issued on September 30, 2010, does identify children's health as a top priority for the agency. EPA discusses children and other disproportionately exposed and affected groups, including low-income, minority, and indigenous populations, which require more explicit consideration in EPA's chemical risk assessments and management actions under its goal of ensuring the safety of chemicals and preventing pollution. In addition, the agency more specifically discusses how it plans to address children's health in its Cross-Cutting Strategy on Environmental Justice and Children's Health, which describes the following objectives:[41]

- Implement the nation's environmental laws in its regulatory capacity through use of the best science and environmental monitoring data to address environmental justice and children's health considerations at each stage of the regulation development process.

- Develop and use environmental and public health indicators to measure improvements in environmental conditions and health in disproportionately impacted communities and among vulnerable age groups.

- Take into account disproportionately impacted, overburdened populations and vulnerable age groups and encourage the use of "green chemistry" to spur the development of safer chemicals and production processes in its work on safe management of pesticides and industrial chemicals.

- Apply the best scientific methods to assess the potential for disproportionate exposures and health impacts resulting from

---

[40]GAO-10-205.

[41]In its strategic plan, EPA discusses a set of cross-cutting strategies it developed that are to achieve the mission outcomes articulated under its five strategic goals.

environmental hazards on minority, and other vulnerable populations.

- Engage communities fully in its work to protect human health and the environment, working to address critical issues affecting children's health and disproportionately impacted, overburdened populations.

- Work with other federal agencies to engage communities and coordinate funding and technical support for efforts to build healthy, sustainable, and green neighborhoods, and work with residents to promote equitable development.

According to the strategic plan, EPA will develop an annual action plan for each year of the strategic plan that lists specific actions and related targets the agency will take in carrying out the operating principles in the cross-cutting strategy. For example, in its 2011 annual action plan in helping to better manage pesticides and industrial chemicals, EPA committed to identifying 5 to 10 priority chemical hazards to children's health by April 2011. The agency also committed in the action plan to consulting with the CHPAC to develop children's health criteria for identifying chemicals for assessment and action under TSCA. According to EPA's 2011 action plan status report, both actions have been completed.

EPA Has Reevaluated and Updated the Mission of the Office of Children's Health Protection and Its Director

In our January 2010 report, we recommended that EPA reevaluate the mission of OCHP and its Director to make the office "an agency-wide champion" for children's environmental health. EPA reorganized the Administrator's Office, including OCHP, in July 2010. To increase OCHP's focus on children's health, EPA moved the Office of Aging and the Environmental Education Division that had been located in the office. In addition, EPA created within OCHP the Regulatory Support and Science Policy Division to work with regulations and science, as well as the Program Implementation and Coordination Division to conduct coordination and outreach with program and regional offices.[42] Prior to this reorganization, OCHP's mission was broader including a focus on aging as well as environmental education.[43] The OCHP Director told us

---

[42]Previously, OCHP was divided into four areas: (1) outreach and partnerships; (2) regulations, economics, data analysis; (3) science; and (4) aging initiative.

[43]OCHP's prior mission was to "make the health protection of children and the aging a fundamental goal of public health and environmental protection in the United States and around the world."

GAO-13-254 EPA Children's Health

that, prior to the reorganization, OCHP focused more on science policy than on regulatory activities. The reorganization narrowed the mission and as noted in OCHP's fiscal 2011-2013 strategic plan, the office's mission is to ensure that EPA actions and programs further the protection of children's environmental health.

The EPA Administrator assigned new responsibilities to OCHP in the February 2010 memorandum to EPA staff. According to the memorandum, OCHP is directed to take the lead in ensuring that program and regional offices are successful in their children's health efforts; in addition, the memo indicates that the OCHP Director will be the main point-of-contact to assist program and regional offices in making children's environmental health a priority in all agency programs and actions. OCHP staff reported that the Director now participates in senior-level meetings, including regulatory update meetings with the Deputy Administrator, quarterly meetings with regional managers, and attends senior policy meetings and program updates.

EPA Is Proactively Using the Children's Health Protection Advisory Committee

In our January 2010 report, we recommended that EPA use CHPAC proactively as a mechanism for providing advice on regulations, programs, plans, or other issues. EPA is using CHPAC as we recommended. For example, in March 2012, EPA sought advice from CHPAC in developing lead regulations and in coordinating agency programs to prevent childhood lead exposure. Additionally, at the request of the OCHP Director, CHPAC assisted in developing information about asthma disparities among racial and ethnic groups for EPA to use as part of its work on the President's Task Force on Environmental Health Risks and Safety Risks to Children, which was established in 1997 and charged with recommending strategies for protecting children's environmental health and safety. In May 2012, the task force published the *Coordinated Federal Action Plan to Reduce Racial and Ethnic Asthma Disparities*.

Furthermore, EPA program offices have also worked more closely with CHPAC on a number of issues related to children's heath since we issued our January 2010 report, according to CHPAC's Co-Chair. For example, EPA's Office of Air and Radiation provided a briefing to CHPAC on indoor air quality to help the committee identify priority areas. CHPAC's

Designated Federal Officer (DFO)[44] also works with other federal advisory committees, such as EPA's Clean Air Scientific Advisory Committee and the Science Advisory Board on other issues to coordinate as needed.

EPA Is Consistently Participating in Key Interagency Organizations Initiated Under Executive Order 13045

In our January 2010 report, we found that EPA's involvement in two organizations authorized by Executive Order 13045 had not been consistent over the years. These organizations included the Federal Interagency Forum on Child and Family Statistics (Forum), a working group of 22 federal agencies that collect, analyze, and report data on conditions and trends in issues related to child and family well-being and the previously mentioned President's Task Force. As a result, we recommended that EPA ensure participation, to the fullest extent possible, by OCHP or other key EPA officials in these interagency organizations.

OCHP officials told us they have been active participants in the Forum by helping to prepare statistical data and descriptive text on children's well-being, such as lead levels in the blood of children that are included in the Forum's biennial publications: *America's Children* (2011) and *America's Children in Brief* (2010). Additionally, an OCHP official is a member of the Forum's reporting committee, which works on a number of issues involved in the creation of these reports, and has the responsibility to write and edit the Physical Environment and Safety section of *America's Children in Brief*. OCHP also contributed to the 2012 edition of *America's Children in Brief: Key National Indicators of Well-Being* and is working on the 2013 edition of *America's Children*.

OCHP officials also told us that they have had a major role in reinvigorating the President's Task Force Steering Committee. The Task Force officially expired in 2005. Although the task force has not been officially reauthorized, EPA and other agencies that were members of the task force have been participating in various efforts to address children's health concerns since January 2010.[45] For example, OCHP's Director has served as the Co-Chair of the Task Force that, among other things,

---

[44]A DFO is a required position for all committees established under the Federal Advisory Committee Act (FACA). The DFO may chair each advisory committee meeting, approve agendas and maintain records, among other duties.

[45]According to EPA officials, the decision to reinvigorate the task force was announced in January 2010 in Washington, D.C., and was a result of talks between EPA, HHS, and the Executive Council on Environmental Quality.

addresses healthy homes, chemical exposures, and asthma disparities. For example, the task force held a workshop on asthma disparities in December 2010 and, as we stated previously, in May 2012, published the *Coordinated Federal Action Plan to Reduce Racial and Ethnic Asthma Disparities*. OCHP officials said the office also played a major role in the task force's 2012 efforts to coordinate federal action on lead exposure.

EPA Has Taken Steps to Address Three Recommendations Supporting Children's Health but Has Not Fully Implemented Them

The agency has taken some steps to address the three remaining recommendations from our January 2010 report but has not fully implemented them.

Program Offices Do Not Consistently Identify Actions Involving Children's Health in EPA's Regulatory Tracking System

In our January 2010 report, we found that EPA could not be assured that the agency had thoroughly addressed risks to infants and children because it neither systematically evaluated nor consistently documented how the agency considered children's health risks in rulemaking. As a result, we recommended that the agency strengthen the data system that identifies and tracks development of rulemakings and other actions to ensure they comply with the 1995 policy on evaluating health risks to children. Since the issuance of our January 2010 report, EPA has taken some actions to strengthen its data system called ADP Tracker by, among other things, developing more targeted screening questions for rule writers regarding the effects on children's health of rulemakings and other actions. Specifically, EPA added two questions for rule writers to complete to help identify actions potentially involving children's health when initiating a new workgroup addressing matters that may be appropriate for OCHP staff participation (see fig. 3 for the screening questions). According to Office of Policy officials, OCHP is one of a few EPA offices that has specific questions in ADP Tracker to assist its work. The officials said that these screening questions are an important tool to inform OCHP when a rulemaking is being initiated that may affect children's health issues, so that OCHP may decide whether to become involved and assign resources.

Figure 3: Questions Used to Help Identity Actions Potentially Involving Children's Health

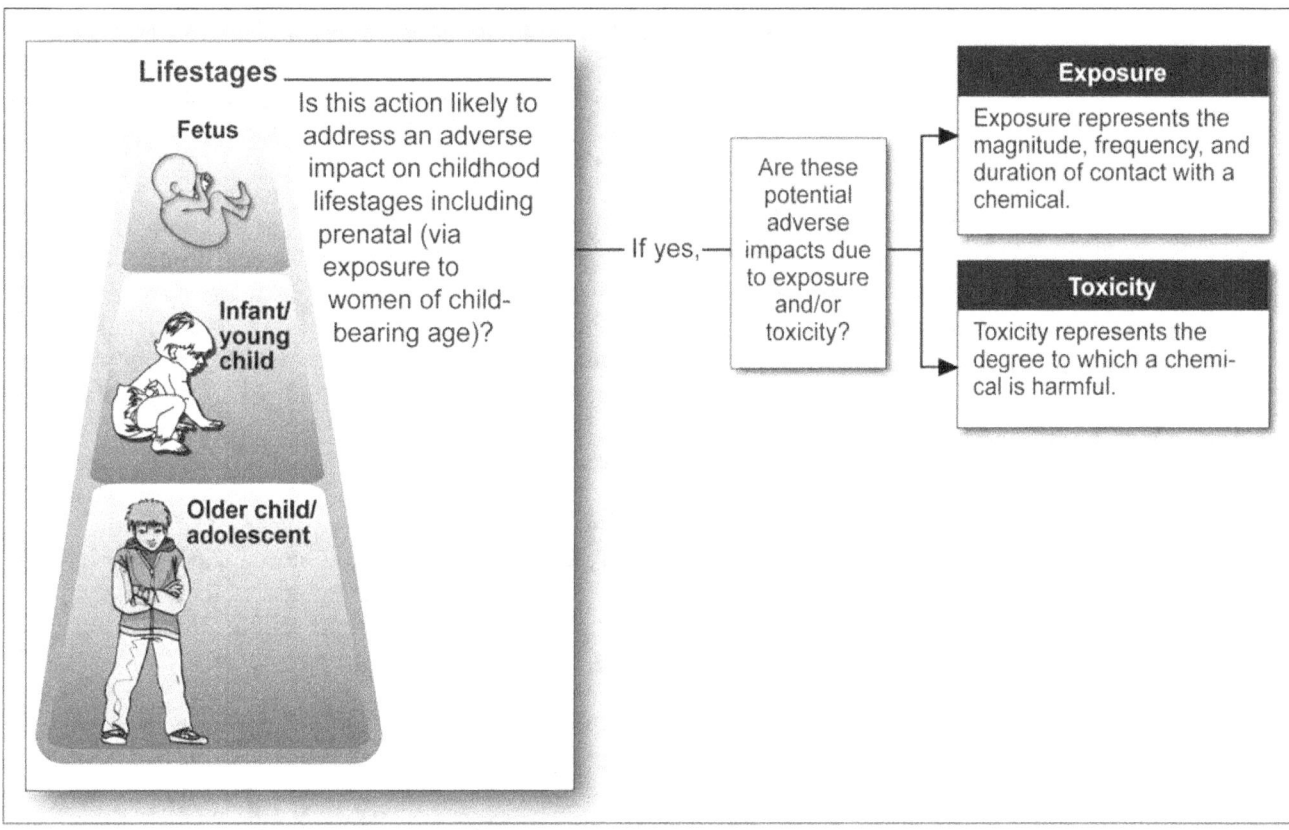

Sources: EPA, Art Explosion (images), and GAO.

However, OCHP cannot rely on these questions to consistently identify workgroups that are addressing matters that may be appropriate for OCHP staff participation because program offices' rule writers have not consistently identified workgroup actions involving children's health in ADP Tracker through the screening questions. A 2011 OCHP analysis has shown that, in some cases, the screening questions may not have been clearly understood by rule writers and left blank and, in other cases, rule writers may not have had the level of expertise necessary to complete the screening questions accurately. OCHP officials said that the 2011 analysis showed that, in some cases, rule writers incorrectly indicated that a proposed action had no children's health implications. According to an OCHP official, one rule writer on a workgroup drafting a rule on national emission standards for hazardous air pollutants did not check "yes" in the ADP Tracker to indicate that the rule would impact children's health until after discussing the issue with OCHP officials. The misunderstanding stemmed from the requirements in the Clean Air Act regarding technology-based standards. Even though the workgroup did perform analyses of the impacts of the rule to children, because the rule was primarily a technology-based mercury reduction standard other factors, including health implications for children, could not be considered when setting the standard. EPA offers training on how to consider children's health issues in the ADP, but according to Office of Policy officials this training is not required for rule writers to understand how to respond to the screening questions related to children's health. According to Office of Policy officials, rule writers represent a range of experiences with some having a broad understanding of children's health issues, while others have very little; as a result, training is left to the discretion of each rule writer. OCHP officials acknowledged that rule writers may not have all the information necessary early on in the rulemaking process to determine whether an action has children's health implications and, because they may have a limited understanding of how to address the screening question, they might not initially answer them. However, as one OCHP official noted, rule writers may revisit the screening questions at another point in the ADP, but they do not always do so for a variety of reasons, including limited data about the potential effect on children of what the rule is addressing as well as competing priorities.

OCHP officials told us that because of the issues with the screening questions in ADP Tracker identified in the 2011 analysis, they are using an alternative method—manually reviewing monthly tiering reports prepared by EPA's Regulatory Steering Committee that list new regulations being developed by program offices, which would be unnecessary if answers to the screening questions were reliable.[46] OCHP officials said the most effective way to ensure health risks to children are being assessed is to have OCHP staff participate in regulatory workgroups early in rulemaking activities. To become involved early in a rulemaking process, OCHP officials said they must be aware of a rulemaking at or near its initiation and have information on the extent to which the rulemaking could involve consideration of children's health effects.

---

[46]Office of Policy officials noted that these monthly reports are reviewed throughout the agency by various offices to identify other offices' relevant rulemakings. These reviews, according to Office of Policy officials, are generally the basis for potentially interested offices to make their initial decisions about whether and how to participate in an action.

In addition to difficulties in reliably identifying actions that involve children's health, EPA does not have a specific process for the program office leading a regulatory workgroup to document compliance with the 1995 children's health policy, which calls for certain steps regarding children's risks when a risk assessment is being conducted for a rulemaking. For example, in our May 2011 report on EPA's implementation of SDWA requirements,[47] we found that, for certain regulatory actions, EPA did not develop a child-specific risk assessment or document why one was not done. In that report, we found that the Office of Water had not developed separate children's risk assessments when developing the 2008 regulatory determinations. Office of Water officials said that they believed their evaluation of the health risks of contaminants took into account sensitive subpopulations, including children, as required by the act. As we reported, EPA's 2008 regulatory determination documentation did not explain how or whether the agency determined that a separate risk assessment for children was not warranted. EPA staff involved in the 2008 regulatory determination told us they were aware of EPA guidance for considering children's health but were unaware of the 1995 policy.

When we asked for documentation on whether child-specific risk assessments were being conducted for current actions, as required by the 1995 policy, EPA was not able to provide this information. Officials from OCHP and the Office of Policy agreed that compliance with the 1995 policy is not being documented in ADP Tracker. They suggested that this documentation could occur at different stages of the ADP. Officials from OCHP and the Office of Policy said that one possible way to document whether a risk assessment was or was not being conducted would be in the development of the analytical blueprint during the ADP, which establishes what analyses will be done to support the proposed rule. This would show that a risk assessment could be expected as part of the rule package or that none was necessary. Another option suggested by the Office of Policy official would be to document whether a child-specific risk assessment was completed near the end of the ADP at the Final Agency Review step, which occurs before the action package is sent to OMB or signed by the Administrator.

---

[47]GAO, *Safe Drinking Water Act: EPA Should Improve Implementation of Requirements on Whether to Regulate Additional Contaminants*, GAO-11-254 (Washington, D.C.: May 27, 2011).

EPA Has Reevaluated Its 1995 Children's Health Policy and Believes It Is Adequate for Ensuring Consistency with New Scientific Research

In our January 2010 report, we recommended that EPA reevaluate its 1995 policy to ensure that it is consistent with new scientific research demonstrating the risks childhood exposures can have for developing disease later in life. As we stated earlier, the 1995 policy directs EPA staff to consistently and explicitly consider risks to infants and children as a part of risk assessments generated during its decision-making processes— or state clearly why it did not—in rulemakings and when setting standards to protect public health and the environment.

OCHP has updated various guidance documents since 1995 to emphasize the use of the best available science regarding children's health risks. The OCHP Director told us that EPA had not updated the 1995 policy because doing so would be resource intensive, taking away from the office's involvement in regulatory and other actions, and becoming a strain on limited staff. OCHP officials stated that the intent of the 1995 policy is to include all of the latest advances in children's health as the science continues to evolve and noted that, while the 1995 policy has not been updated, other relevant guidance documents have been brought up to date to ensure that current science is used to achieve the general policy.[48] Officials also stated that the February 2010 memo from the Administrator discusses using the "best available research and data" and "best science" regarding children's health risks. While OCHP officials said that the 1995 policy is still sufficient, senior staff from OCHP acknowledged that a reaffirmation of the 1995 policy would help clarify that the intent of the 1995 policy is to include the latest advances in science, elevate the importance of using applicable guidance, and would reiterate EPA's commitment to protecting children's health. We agree that such a reaffirmation would help clarify the intent of the policy but believe our prior recommendation still has merit.

---

[48]The following guidance documents address children's health considerations and reference the links between early life exposures and disease later in life: *2005 Supplemental Guidance for Assessing Susceptibility from Early-Life Exposures to Carcinogens*; 2006 *Guidance for Selecting Age Groups for Monitoring and Assessing Childhood Exposure to Environmental Contaminants*; 2006 *Framework for Assessing Heath Risks of Environmental Exposures to Children,* and EPA's Office of Research and Development's 2008 *Child-Specific Exposure Factors Handbook.*

EPA Has Not Established Key Children's Health Staff within Program and Regional Offices to Coordinate with OCHP

In our January 2010 report, we recommended that EPA establish key environmental health staff within each program and regional office, with linkages to OCHP, to improve cross-agency implementation of revised priorities and goals and ensure coordination and communication among EPA's program offices. EPA has designated 10 regional school coordinators to improve coordination in the regions, but it has not established an OCHP liaison in each program office. The regional school coordinators work on all EPA programs within their respective regions that affect schools and school districts as well as with states and school professionals; they also address requirements for indoor air quality, chemicals used in the classroom, and encourage Energy Star energy efficiency activities, efforts to reduce accidental exposures to chemicals, improvements to outdoor air quality, recycling, community development, and proper siting of schools. The official said an OCHP liaison works with the regional school coordinators and holds monthly conference calls to coordinate these efforts. The OCHP liaison is also to coordinate with regions and program offices to ensure schools goals are met and measures are established. Similarly, the official said, a children's environmental health protection coordinator within OCHP works with the 10 regional children's environmental health coordinators to ensure that regional activities are consistent with EPA strategic plans and goals in settings other than schools, such as child-care facilities.

According to OCHP staff, the children's environmental health coordinators also assist other constituencies like health care providers, parents, community leaders, and state and local officials addressing particular health issues relevant to children, such as asthma and lead exposure. The OCHP Director also has quarterly conference calls with regional senior-level managers with children's health responsibilities to facilitate information sharing between OCHP and the regions. According to OCHP staff, the OCHP Director also attends regulatory update meetings with EPA's Deputy Administrator and holds periodic conference calls with senior-level program staff when the need arises. When we asked why EPA has not established an OCHP liaison in each program office, the OCHP Director stated that there is ample communication between OCHP and top program officials with respect to children's health protection. In addition, the OCHP Director said that the periodic conference calls and other communication efforts are sufficient in making children's health a focus in program offices and said that instituting a children's health liaison in each program office is not necessary, but it may offer value. We agree that OCHP has increased communication at the regional level; however, we continue to believe that a liaison is needed in program offices because while communication occurs where OCHP is involved in regulatory workgroups, information sharing is often lacking in other circumstances.

OCHP Has Increased Its Role to Ensure That Most EPA Program Offices Consider Children's Health Protection in Their Regulatory Activities

OCHP has increased its role to ensure that most EPA's program offices consider children's health protection in their regulatory activities. In the Administrator's February 2010 memorandum, OCHP was directed to ensure that all program offices are successful in their efforts to protect children's health. As such, OCHP has played a greater role in program offices' development of selected regulations that potentially affect children's health, since the office's 2010 reorganization. OCHP has been involved in regulations that impact children's health under several major environmental statutes, including the SDWA and FFDCA that include specific children's health language. For example, OCHP has been more actively involved in determining drinking water program standards and other regulatory actions, including regulatory determinations, under SDWA. However, officials told us that the office has no regular involvement in and limited familiarity with OPP's ongoing decision-making processes associated with the setting of individual tolerance levels in foods conducted under FFDCA.

OCHP Has Played a Greater Role in Program Offices' Development of Selected Regulations That Potentially Affect Children's Health

Consistent with the direction in the EPA Administrator's February 2010 memorandum, OCHP is to take the lead in ensuring that the programs and regions are successful in their efforts to protect children's health. Since the reorganization of the office in 2010, OCHP has been involved in more regulatory workgroups using the ADP, thereby playing a greater supporting role in program offices' development of rules and regulations that could potentially affect children's health. OCHP primarily supports EPA program offices during the ADP, such as the Office of Air and the Office of Water, by providing a children's health perspective to regulatory workgroups that are responsible for developing EPA actions, rules, and regulations. The OCHP Director told us that OCHP was participating in more regulatory workgroups than at any time in the history of the office to reflect the priorities of the Administrator, which are consistent with the agency's strategic plan. According to ADP guidance, there are several ways that OCHP can get involved in workgroups that are developing regulations that could potentially affect children's health. For example, the program office with lead responsibility for developing an EPA action, rule, or regulation could ask OCHP to participate on a workgroup typically at the initial stages of the ADP. OCHP could also request to participate on the workgroup, as an official member or as an unofficial advisor, if OCHP believes that children's health issues are involved.[49] According to OCHP officials, while participating on a workgroup, OCHP has the opportunity to provide input in the development of regulations. OCHP also can raise concerns with a proposed regulation at the final review stage, but officials from EPA's Office of Policy and OCHP said that OCHP generally attempts to work out problems before they reach this point.

In fiscal year 2011, of the 106 new or ongoing regulations listed in EPA's publicly available regulatory tracking system,[50] 31 were identified by program offices as having a potential impact on children's health. Of those 31 regulations, OCHP officials told us they participated in workgroups involved in the development of 21 because they felt these were the highest priority actions for children's health. To assist in determining whether workgroups adequately considered children's health concerns, OCHP developed factors to measure whether ongoing workgroups were fully responsive to children's health matters. The factors[51] include information, such as whether the workgroup sufficiently addressed comments from OCHP staff; the workgroup reviewed child-specific literature, evaluated child-specific hazards and/or exposures, and selected appropriate child-specific risk management options; and whether OCHP staff participated in the workgroup. OCHP officials said that the determination as to whether a workgroup has been responsive to these factors is based on the professional judgment and experience of the OCHP staff member who serves on the workgroup. When an OCHP staff member did not serve on a workgroup, OCHP contacted the program office to ascertain how responsive the workgroup was to children's health concerns based on the factors described above. According to OCHP's

---

[49]For actions that are conducted under the ADP, OCHP can use the ADP Tracker to identify rules flagged as potentially implicating children's health, and then indicate it wishes to participate on the workgroup. However, as we are reporting, the data in ADP Tracker may not be complete. In addition, OCHP also has access to other databases that list rules EPA is working on, and has regular meetings with the Office of Policy to discuss rules and other topics of interest.

[50]This publicly available system called Reg DAART, includes a subset of information from ADP Tracker, which is EPA's internal tracking system.

[51]OCHP officials provided us with a list of six possible factors, which they refer to as criteria, including whether child-specific scientific literature was reviewed, but not all criteria are applicable to all actions.

assessment, agency officials estimated that 20 of the 31 workgroups were fully responsive to children's health concerns at the time of their assessment, and 11 were not.[52] This OCHP assessment was a subjective review to address a goal in the OCHP strategic plan to provide the office with a perspective on the responsiveness of actions at a point during the ongoing ADP. While program offices did not have an opportunity to assess OCHP's analysis, OCHP used the results to compare the success of the groups they participated in with those they did not. OCHP officials said that their analysis indicated workgroups were more likely to be responsive to children's health concerns when an OCHP staff member serves on the workgroup. For a listing of these actions, see appendix IV.

Of the 31 regulatory workgroups involved with actions identified as having potential impact on children's health, we reviewed the 6 that had finalized rules at the time of our analysis.[53] We interviewed EPA program officials about OCHP's role and effectiveness on the 6 workgroups we reviewed. We also interviewed OCHP staff members who served on 4 of the 6 workgroups. In some cases, OCHP staff members described OCHP's contribution as limited because of the highly technical nature of the rule being considered or because OCHP joined the workgroup too late in the ADP.

In addition to workgroup participants, we also spoke with officials from several key program offices, including from the offices of Air, Water, Chemical Safety and Pollution Prevention, and Solid Waste and Emergency Response. These officials had positive comments about OCHP staff members' contribution to their workgroups but said that they do not consistently utilize OCHP staff on their workgroups during the rulemaking process. For example, an official from one program office noted that OCHP does not have enough staff to participate in all of that office's workgroups dealing with children's health matters. According to OCHP officials, tracking the early steps of the rulemaking process manually through monthly tiering reports, as discussed earlier, is OCHP's

---

[52]OCHP served on 3 of the 11 workgroups. For the remaining 8, OCHP consulted with workgroup chairs in making their assessment for the workgroups responsiveness to children's health.

[53]Our analysis of the 6 workgroups that addressed final rules includes 2 of the 11 workgroups that EPA found to be not fully responsive to children's health issues. Of the 2 that were not fully responsive, OCHP served on one of them, which involved the efficiency of heavy duty vehicles to reduce greenhouse gas emissions.

current approach for identifying and prioritizing workgroups to join as early as possible, as they do not have adequate resources to join every workgroup that may involve children's health matters.[54]

OCHP Has Played a More Active Role in Determining Drinking Water Standards under SDWA since 2010

According to OCHP officials, OCHP began playing a more active role in determining drinking water standards under SDWA and other regulatory actions in 2010, after the Administrator's memo was released.[55] OCHP staff members said that they have participated on workgroups associated with the forthcoming proposal for a drinking water standard for perchlorate—a naturally occurring and man-made chemical that may adversely affect the functioning of the thyroid gland, which produces hormones critical to the normal development and growth of fetuses, infants, and children. The perchlorate standard is scheduled to be proposed in December 2013, according to EPA officials.[56] OCHP staff members also told us they have participated on the workgroups tasked with developing the contaminant candidate list under SDWA and determining whether selected chemicals on the list should be regulated.[57] According to an OCHP official, OCHP staff members have also been involved with developing other rules promulgated by the Office of Water, including revisions to two national drinking water standards. This coordination between the Office of Water and OCHP represents an improvement to what we reported in our May 2011 report,[58] where we found that relevant EPA staff, including staff from OCHP, had limited input in the preliminary regulatory determination for perchlorate. In our 2011 report, we found that, by excluding relevant EPA offices, such as OCHP from a more participatory role, the agency did not avail itself of the expertise that resides in those offices. Instead, we determined that EPA

---

[54]In addition to its manual review of monthly tiering reports, OCHP also reviews the results of screening questions in ADP Tracker to confirm that OCHP has identified relevant workgroups for its participation.

[55]An OCHP official noted that the office began participating on more workgroups for drinking water regulations and standards in March 2010.

[56]EPA, Drinking Water: Regulatory Determination on Perchlorate, 76 Fed. Reg. 7762 (Feb. 11, 2011) available at https://federalregister.gov/a/2011-2603.

[57]As stated earlier, SDWA requires that EPA identify and publish a list every 5 years of unregulated contaminants that may require regulation, called the contaminant candidate list.

[58]GAO-11-254.

relied on the assessment of a small group of high-level management officials in making its 2008 preliminary determination not to regulate perchlorate. In February 2011, EPA reversed its 2008 preliminary decision and decided to regulate perchlorate.

ADP guidance indicates that representatives from any interested program office, such as OCHP, can participate on regulatory workgroups, such as those led by the Office of Water. Office of Water officials we interviewed said that OCHP staff often serve on regulatory workgroups when the topics are pertinent to children's health. The OCHP officials we spoke with confirmed that OCHP staff members have participated on numerous regulatory workgroups initiated by the Office of Water including those developing National Primary Drinking Water Regulations.[59] For example, OCHP staff members serve on the workgroup addressing revisions to the lead and copper rule and served on the workgroup addressing revisions to the Total Coliform Rule.[60]

---

[59]National Primary Drinking Water Regulations or primary standards are legally enforceable standards that apply to public water systems. Primary standards protect public health by limiting the levels of contaminants in drinking water or imposing treatment technique requirements.

[60]National Primary Drinking Water Regulations for Lead and Copper: Regulatory Revisions (and National Primary Drinking Water Regulations: Revision to the Total Coliform Rule). According to EPA's December 2012 fact sheet, the Total Coliform Rule is intended to improve public health protection by reducing fecal pathogens to minimal levels through control of total coliform bacteria, including fecal coliform.

OCHP Has Had No Regular Involvement in Reviewing the Tolerance Decisions for Pesticide Residues on Foods

Because OPP does not follow the ADP for pesticide tolerance decisions, OCHP, as well as other program offices, are typically not involved in tolerance decisions[61] for pesticide residues on processed and raw foods. In addition, OCHP officials told us they do not track OPP's decisions noting that OPP does not identify pesticide tolerance decisions with children's health implications that would potentially enable OCHP to be involved.[62] As such, OCHP is not informed about changes OPP makes to margins of safety for infants and children.[63] OPP generally publishes explanations for its decisions to lower safety factors in the *Federal Register*, some of which have been described by some experts from academia and industry as complex or incomplete.

OCHP Is Not Involved in Pesticide Tolerance Decisions

Although pesticide tolerance decisions can greatly affect children's health, OCHP is not involved in such decisions. Office of Policy officials explained that these decisions have never been conducted under the ADP, which could involve OCHP and the other program offices. There are several reasons why this is the case. First, officials said that the ADP generally applies to actions that are prompted by EPA. According to officials, tolerance decision processes are not generally prompted by EPA; instead, they are in response to submissions, called petitions, received from industry or the public.[64] Further, Office of Policy officials stated that these decisions are not signed by the Administrator and do not appear in the Regulatory Agenda—a long-standing method of handling tolerance decisions that has been agreed to by the Administrator of EPA and the Administrator of OMB's Office of Information and Regulatory

---

[61]As stated earlier, for purposes of this report, we refer to "tolerance decisions" as including not only the establishment or revision of a tolerance but also decisions to grant an exemption from the requirement for a tolerance. In addition, we refer to tolerance decisions in all contexts, which may include situations such as where a tolerance is established or reviewed as part of a pesticide registration or reregistration or a new use application, in response to a petition, or others.

[62]OPP posts its work plans on the EPA website. OCHP could review them to determine if it should get involved in pesticide registration and tolerance decisions. However, OCHP officials told us that the office has limited resources to devote to this activity and that the information included in these public documents does not always contain sufficient information to address children's health priorities.

[63]According to EPA, In the late 1990s, OCHP had early involvement in establishing the framework for the risk assessment process that the OPP program continues to use for making tolerance decisions today.

[64]Office of Policy officials also noted that there are statutory time frames applicable to certain steps, such as determining tolerance petitions are complete.

Affairs.[65] OPP officials told us they publish more than 10000 *Federal Register* documents each year (e.g., notice of filings and final rules) that are related to tolerance decisions; this high frequency of actions is another reason OPP officials cited for why their office does not use the ADP process as it needs efficient procedures to handle tolerance decisions.[66] The Pesticide Registration Improvements Extension Act imposes specific deadlines on EPA for pending applications for pesticide actions and, according to officials, the high frequency of actions would impede the agency's ability to adhere to these time frames.

In a written response to GAO, OPP officials also said that EPA decision making for tolerance decisions is relatively straightforward, generally receives few public comments, has resulted in "very few" lawsuits, and does not need an ADP workgroup to develop and evaluate regulatory options.[67] OPP officials also referred to language commonly found in EPA's Semi-Annual Regulatory Agendas that describes pesticide tolerances as routine actions.[68] However, in a separate written response to GAO, OPP officials noted that such decisions can be particularly complex. Given the required evaluation of numerous toxicity databases and exposure analyses, among other assessments that go into tolerance decisions, it is unclear how such decisions could be routine in nature.

As we stated earlier, the Administrator directs OCHP to take the lead in ensuring that all EPA programs are successful in their efforts to protect children's health. Since OPP does not participate in the ADP or any other collaborative process for pesticide tolerance decisions, and some of these

---

[65]Under Executive Order 12866, the Office of Information and Regulatory Affairs reviews certain agency draft regulations—generally those that are economically or otherwise significant—before publication. According to the White House website, the office's review serves to ensure adequate interagency review of draft rules, so that agencies coordinate their rules with other agencies to avoid inconsistent, incompatible, or duplicative policies.

[66]For comparison purposes, Office of Policy officials noted that there are approximately 100 new actions tiered for the agency annually in the ADP.

[67]EPA stated that there have been only five legal challenges to EPA tolerance decisions while there have been more than ten thousand tolerance decisions made since passage of the FQPA.

[68]See, for example, EPA, Regulatory Agenda, 54 Fed. Reg. 45,272 (Oct. 30, 1989) ("the listings exclude ...routine actions (such as pesticide tolerances)"). Officials noted that this language has been used for more than 2 decades and still appears in every Semi-Annual Regulatory Agenda.

decisions may have an impact on children's health, OCHP and OPP are not operating consistently with the direction laid out in the memorandum.

OCHP Is not Involved in Changes to Pesticide Tolerance Margins of Safety

OPP is primarily responsible for implementing the requirements of FFDCA with respect to tolerances and generally has not coordinated tolerance decisions with OCHP or with other EPA offices.[69] OPP officials do not identify pesticide tolerance decisions with children's health implications for OCHP involvement, nor do OCHP officials track OPP's workplans for pesticide registrations or OPP's decisions published in the *Federal Register*.

From 1996 to 2012, OPP made pesticide tolerance decisions for 412 pesticides and, in 308 or 75 percent of the cases, OPP applied a lower safety factor than the default 10-fold margin of safety for infants and children established by FQPA. OCHP was not involved in any of these decisions, even with the direction by the Administrator's 2010 memorandum indicating that it should take the lead in ensuring that EPA programs are successful in their efforts to protect children's health. To make pesticide tolerance decisions, OPP conducts the needed analyses and assessments with its technical and policy/regulatory staff, in consultation with the Office of General Counsel, and it has developed a data set that tracks its decisions regarding the use of the FQPA safety factor over time.[70] As shown in figure 4, OPP applied a 1-fold or 3-fold safety factor, in 308 instances, or 75 percent of the time.[71] OPP retained

---

[69]EPA officials noted that the agency's Office of General Counsel reviews most tolerance decisions, among other decision documents.

[70]The information provided reflects the highest FQPA safety factor for a pesticide when there are different safety factors addressing various exposure scenarios for a given pesticide. In some instances, EPA may apply different FQPA safety factors to different exposure scenarios, depending on the reliability of available data for those scenarios.

[71]Data on safety factor decisions for this period were compiled and provided by OPP and report the most current and highest OPP-applied safety factor for each pesticide. The data do not count all the tolerances for each pesticide, because for each pesticide there may be multiple tolerances for multiple food products. The data also do not capture instances where a pesticide might have initially been assigned a 10-fold safety factor that was later reduced, such as after additional studies were completed. In less than 1 percent of the cases, EPA applied a safety factor that was an outlier and did not fit into the 1-fold, 3-fold, 10-fold, or 30-fold safety factor category. In 3 percent of the cases, EPA applied a safety factor greater than the default 10-fold safety factor.

the default 10-fold safety factor established by FQPA for less than one-quarter of the pesticides for which it made tolerance decisions.[72]

Figure 4: EPA Summary of Pesticides with Safety Factor Decisions from 1996 to 2012

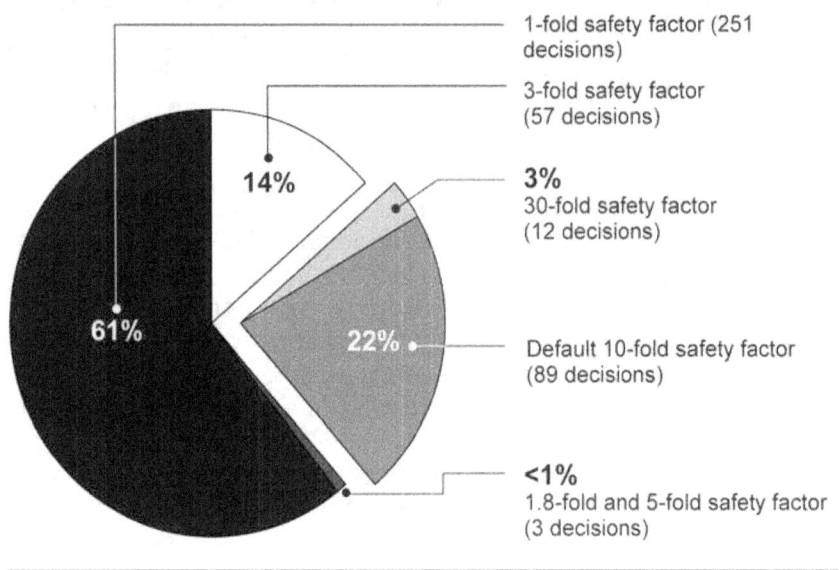

1-fold safety factor (251 decisions)

3-fold safety factor (57 decisions)

3%
30-fold safety factor (12 decisions)

Default 10-fold safety factor (89 decisions)

<1%
1.8-fold and 5-fold safety factor (3 decisions)

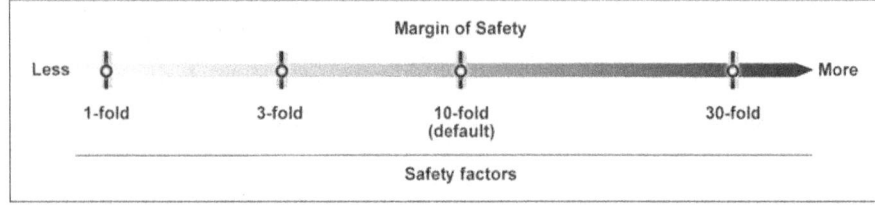

Source: GAO analysis of EPA data.

Note: This figure represents 412 safety factor decisions made by EPA from 1996 through 2012. EPA determines the safety factor based on data completeness and children's susceptibility and applies the selected safety factor to its calculations during risk assessments to determine the pesticide chemical residue allowed on raw and processed foods. A lower safety factor reflects less uncertainty about data completeness and fewer unaddressed concerns about children's susceptibility whereas a higher safety factor denotes more uncertainty regarding these factors. FFDCA requires that, when setting a tolerance level for pesticides, EPA is to assess risks to infants and children and apply an additional 10-fold margin of safety for the pesticide chemical residue and other sources of exposure to take into

[72]Similarly, in September 2000, we reported that OPP applied the 10-fold safety factor in 20 percent of the 105 safety factor decisions as of the end of March 2000 and a safety factor greater than 10-fold in 5 percent of the decisions. See GAO, *Children and Pesticides: New Approach to Considering Risk is Partly in Place*, GAO/HEHS-00-175 (Washington, D.C.: Sept. 11, 2000).

account potential pre-and postnatal toxicity and other factors. The act provides the Administrator of EPA with the authority to use a different margin of safety for a pesticide chemical residue if, on the basis of reliable data, such a margin would be safe for infants and children.

OPP officials told us that the agency bases the decisions to lower the FQPA safety factor on data they find reliable that demonstrate that a lower FQPA safety factor is protective of infants and children. OPP's approach to analyzing the FQPA safety factor is to consider three areas of review: (1) completeness of the toxicity database—whether all the required toxicity studies on the pesticide have been submitted; (2) completeness of exposure database—whether the exposure data on the pesticide are complete; and (3) the potential pre- and postnatal sensitivity—whether fetuses and infants may be particularly sensitive to health effects of the pesticide. In explaining its approach, OPP officials stated that they would remove the default FQPA safety factor if the data are complete, and if the pesticide either shows no potential pre- or postnatal toxicity, or the dose level at which any pre- or postnatal toxicity is seen is well-defined. Conversely, OPP officials stated if concerns or uncertainties are raised concerning any of the three reasons (toxicity database, exposure database, pre- and postnatal toxicity), EPA would likely retain an additional safety factor.[73] OPP stated that the rationale for each decision is presented in the *Federal Register* notices and supported by documents in the docket.[74] In appendix V, we include information that OPP officials provided us on the rationale associated with tolerance decisions for 1 year—fiscal year 2011.

Even with the analyses conducted by OPP to support its FQPA safety factor decisions, OCHP recently participated in OPP's review of the tolerance for chlorpyrifos to assure that children's health is being adequately protected.[75] For example, in 2011, external stakeholders noticed that OPP issued for public comment a draft evaluation of the human health risks associated with chlorpyrifos through a *Federal Register* notice. Chlorpyrifos is a pesticide that was discontinued from almost all home use in 2000 and discontinued or limited in certain foods,

---

[73]The size of the additional factor would depend on the degree of uncertainty raised.

[74]According to OPP officials, they have taken public comment on the vast majority of these decisions as part of the office's public participation process for pesticide risk assessments.

[75]EPA stated that there have been few objections, and, as previously noted, only five legal challenges to EPA tolerance decisions since passage of the FQPA.

such as apples, grapes, and tomatoes because of its effect on children's neurological systems. Until the stakeholder brought the matter to OCHP's attention, OCHP did not know that OPP was considering reducing the default safety factor from 10-fold to 1-fold in its determination of the chlorpyrifos tolerance for some foods. OCHP voiced its desire to be involved in the decision-making process so as to ensure children's health risks would be adequately accounted for and reached an agreement with OPP to provide a part-time staff person to work with OPP staff on the chlorpyrifos issue.[76]

OCHP officials noted that, without a process whereby OPP and OCHP can establish procedures for identifying tolerance decisions that could pose a significant risk to children's health, it will be difficult for OCHP to engage in the future on those issues and take the lead in ensuring that programs are successful in their efforts to protect children's health, as articulated in the 2010 Administrator's memorandum. As we reported earlier, relying on relationships with individual officials alone as a means of establishing regular coordination among offices is often incomplete and inefficient.[77] Moreover, these informal relationships could end once personnel move to their next assignments. Without updated, integrated, and comprehensive procedures in place for establishing and maintaining interactions among entities, the overall effectiveness of intra-agency collaboration can be limited.

Industry and Academic Experts' Queried on Pesticide Tolerance Decisions and the Need for OCHP Involvement in Them

We contacted eight experts from academia and industry to discuss OPP's FQPA safety factor decisions and whether there was a need for OCHP's involvement in pesticide tolerance decisions. The experts included academics with expertise in pesticide health effects on children, and industry scientists who are regularly involved in pesticide registrations. Most of the experts we interviewed noted that, based on their past experience in reviewing particular EPA tolerance decisions, some of the evidence that EPA used to support its decisions is considered confidential business information (CBI) and is therefore unavailable for public review. Industry experts confirmed that some data are considered CBI subject to EPA protective regulations and thus are excluded from the docket and

---

[76]OCHP officials told us that the level of effort by OCHP for participating in matters related to chlorpyrifos is not sustainable for other pesticides, given OCHP's limited resources.

[77]See GAO, *National Security: Key Challenges and Solutions to Strengthen Interagency Collaboration*, GAO-10-822T (Washington, D.C.: June 9, 2010).

public disclosure.[78] However, OPP officials stated that CBI data are rarely relied on in making a safety determination and OPP reviews of the tolerance data are publicly available. These reviews contain descriptions of how the study was conducted and what effects were observed in the study as well as EPA's conclusions regarding the studies. One academic expert noted that the absence of a group like OCHP in the pesticide decision-making process is problematic because there is no group outside of OPP, other than the Office of General Counsel, and no children's health constituent group consulted in the process. As a result, OCHP cannot respond to outside groups' concerns regarding pesticide decisions that may impact children's health, although it is directed to be EPA's lead office on children's health matters.

Moreover, the five academic experts, but none of the industry experts, raised some concerns with the clarity of the published explanations for EPA's decision to not use the default safety factor. However all of the industry experts, most of whom have day-to-day involvement in pesticide registrations, stated that the FQPA safety factor decisions were generally what they expected and that OPP's explanations were adequate. The industry experts also agreed that the information supporting EPA's decisions can be difficult to interpret and believed the agency could do a better job of explaining its process and presenting the tolerance information. All of the academic experts we spoke with, most of whom are not directly involved in the pesticide registration process, stated that the information provided to the public can be difficult to fully understand and were surprised by the frequent reductions in the safety factor.[79]

In addition, a 2011 court case addressed concerns that, in a particular instance, the basis for OPP's decision regarding pesticide residues and what safety factor to protect children's health was not adequately

---

[78] OPP provides a summary of its supporting data in the relevant *Federal Register* notice and generally includes its analyses of health and safety studies and exposure data in the docket.

[79] We reported on challenges concerning the clarity and transparency of EPA's development and presentation of information on health effects that may result from exposure to environmental contamination in GAO, *Chemical Assessments: Challenges Remain with EPA's Integrated Risk Information System Program*, GAO-12-42 (Washington, D.C.: Dec. 9, 2011.

explained.[80] In Natural Resources Defense Council (NRDC) v. EPA, the U.S. Court of Appeals for the Second Circuit held that, for a subset of the risk assessments EPA did not provide an explanation of why a children's safety factor of less than the default 10-fold was designed "to take into account potential pre- and postnatal toxicity and completeness of the data with respect to infants and children."[81] The court also held that EPA did not identify reliable data and explain how those data showed that a safety factor of less than the default 10-fold would be safe for infants and children. In 2012, in response to the court's remand, EPA issued another order, which again denied NRDC's challenge to EPA's tolerance decision using the lowered safety factor.[82] While EPA reached the same decision as it had previously—that is, that the reduced (3-fold) safety factor would protect the safety of infants and children, the agency also stated it "now recognizes that the discussion of the FQPA safety factor in its dichlorvos [decision] and orders was less than transparent" and explained that it "used, at times, a form of short-hand that hid rather than elucidated its reasoning on the FQPA safety factor."[83] Accordingly, the order stated that "EPA has provided a revised, more extensive explanation for its position" on the FQPA safety factor. NRDC challenged EPA's revised order, and in

[80] NRDC v. EPA, 658 F.3d 200 (2d Cir. 2011). The court considered EPA's explanations in the interim reregistration decision and two orders respectively denying NRDC's petition and administrative objections. The court's decision, however, directly concerns only one order, and did not vacate or remand the interim reregistration decision. The court denied a second claim and did not address a third claim by NRDC. The order represented a formal decision by EPA in response to objections filed by NRDC under the applicable statutory procedures. NRDC's filing stated two objections to EPA's denial of NRDC's original petition that EPA revoke all dichlorvos tolerances.

[81] The dichlorvos registration and orders involved several distinct risk assessments. The subset of studies implicated here are those that relied on a human study referred to as the Gledhill study, rather than animal studies. 658 F.3d at 217.

[82] EPA, Dichlorvos (DDVP); Order Denying NRDC's Objections on Remand, 77 Fed. Reg. 54,402 (Sept. 5, 2012).

[83] 77 Fed. Reg. at 54,412. Dichlorvos is an insecticide used on crops, animals, and in pest-strips.

June 2013 NRDC and EPA entered a settlement and asked the court to stay the challenge.[84]

While OPP publishes information supporting its pesticide tolerance decisions, many of which relate to children's health, as noted above, the basis for some of these decisions may be difficult to understand, and some information deemed CBI may not be available for public review.[85] Moreover, OCHP has no role in the tolerance decision process, and neither OPP nor OCHP have procedures to inform OCHP of pesticide tolerance decisions that have potential impacts on children's health. With the vast majority of pesticide tolerance decisions being established with safety factors lower than the default safety factor established by FQPA, it is unclear how OCHP is to carry out the mission outlined in the Administrator's 2010 memorandum directing it to ensure that program offices are successful in their efforts to protect children's health.

[84]NRDC filed with the U.S. Court of Appeals for the Second Circuit a petition for review of EPA's 2012 final order. NRDC asserted that in denying its petition for the revocation of the tolerance for dichlorvos, EPA improperly relied on a human health effects study that did not comply with ethical standards in effect at the time, and improperly denied NRDC's hearing request. NRDC asked the court to vacate EPA's 2012 order denying NRDC's objections and evidentiary hearing request, and to prevent EPA from relying on the human study or, in the alternative, order EPA to grant NRDC's hearing request. According to EPA, EPA and NRDC reached a settlement under which EPA agreed to reassess the safe level of exposure to dichlorvos and draft a memorandum explaining its reassessment by May 31, 2014, among other things. According to court documents, if EPA does not perform its obligations under the final settlement agreement by May 31, 2014, NRDC may reinstate the petition for review; conversely, the petition for review shall be subject to dismissal after EPA completes performance of its obligations under the final settlement agreement or if the petition for review is not timely reinstated.

[85]Although not publicly available, according to EPA officials, the actual studies with the raw data can be inspected or viewed as long as the person affirms that he or she will not deliver the data to a foreign or multinational pesticide business.

OCHP Has Worked with External Partners to Leverage Its Resources to Better Protect Children's Health

OCHP has worked extensively with a variety of partners to leverage its resources to better protect children's health. OCHP has, for example, coordinated with federal partners to improve children's environmental health in homes and schools. OCHP also has worked with local, tribal, and public service partners to improve children's environmental health in underserved communities. In addition, OCHP has worked with medical experts to enhance health care providers' knowledge about environmental risks to children.

OCHP Has Coordinated with Federal Partners to Improve Children's Environmental Health in Schools and Homes

OCHP continues to work with a number of federal partners, as well as coordinate internally and with nongovernment partners, to protect children in homes and schools. Specifically, OCHP has helped to develop an integrated strategy, released in February 2013, to encourage healthy home environments for children as a member of the federal Healthy Homes Work Group, which includes members from the Departments of Housing and Urban Development, Health and Human Services, Agriculture, Energy, Labor and the National Institute of Standards and Technology.[86] The strategy, *Advancing Healthy Housing: A Strategy for Action*, includes long-term goals and an integrated website with information on topics, such as poisons and dangerous chemicals, pest control, and child safety. The strategy capitalizes on the collective expertise of the workgroup member agencies by establishing a new vision for addressing health and economic burdens caused by preventable environmental health and safety hazards in the home. The strategy contains five broad goals and priorities in healthy housing for the next 3 to 5 years. Specifically, the strategy calls for (1) establishing federally recognized recommendations for healthy homes, (2) encouraging the adoption of healthy homes recommendations, (3) creating and supporting training and workforce development to address health hazards in housing, (4) educating the public about healthy homes, and (5) supporting research that informs and advances healthy housing in a cost-effective manner. According to the strategy, to achieve these goals, federal partners in the workgroup are urged to coordinate their efforts in a number of activities. For example, to encourage the adoption of healthy

---

[86]The strategy is intended to unify federal action for advancing healthy housing through a comprehensive approach, known as the "healthy homes model." The Healthy Homes Work Group expects the model can be used nationwide to reduce health care costs by promoting better healthy housing conditions.

homes criteria, the workgroup will obtain commitments from member agencies to advance healthy housing, strengthen federal efforts to reduce public health risks in housing, and explore ways to increase funding flexibility across federal and nonfederal programs.

According to EPA officials, the healthy homes website, is expected to be launched in the spring of 2013 by the Department of Housing and Urban Development. The website is intended to be a "one-stop shop," where the public will be able to obtain assistance in creating healthy home environments. The officials said that the website is to consist of a number of interactive functions geared toward providing information to specific users. For example, health topics, such as hazardous household chemicals, integrated pest management, how to identify and mitigate radon, and other items will be tailored for both homeowners and renters. Moreover, according to a draft presentation on the healthy homes website, owners and renters will have the ability to print out personalized home safety checklists by answering a series of questions regarding their homes. Users will also have the ability to identify local resources through a map interface and share information by using social networks links on the website. Users will also have the ability to watch videos and obtain tips on ways to create healthy environments in their homes.

The workgroup's strategy also includes training initiatives, some of which are managed through the National Center for Healthy Housing.[87] According to an OCHP official, the training effort includes approximately 25 courses each year that will reach about 800 participants with EPA funding. The training includes a 2-day course, "Essentials for Healthy Homes Practitioners," and a number of 1-day courses dealing with topics such as pest management, energy efficiency, and other healthy homes topics. The training sessions are offered around the country and will target communities where the need is greatest.

In another initiative, OCHP has worked with federal partners to make schools environmentally safer, particularly with respect to selecting

---

[87]The National Center for Healthy Housing is a nonprofit organization with a staff of 16, including housing, health and environmental professionals with expertise in biostatistics, epidemiology, environmental health, public health, housing policy and industrial hygiene. The center operates the National Healthy Homes Training Center through a cooperative agreement with the CDC and support from the U.S. Department of Housing and Urban Development and EPA. The Training Center is aimed at helping states, cities, and community-based organizations effectively identify and address housing-related hazards.

appropriate school locations and designing state programs to improve environmental health in schools. OCHP has consulted with the Departments of Education and Health and Human Services as well as CHPAC in developing school siting guidelines. OCHP has also collaborated with a number of EPA offices on the school siting guidelines, including EPA's Office of Air and Radiation, Office of Sustainable Communities, and Office of Solid Waste and Emergency Response. These guidelines, which are required under the Energy Independence and Security Act, are voluntary and are designed to help localities, tribes, and the public better understand and appropriately consider environmental and public health factors prior to selecting school locations. They are not intended to replace state, tribal, or local school site or location selection policies or requirements but rather to assist local school districts and community members in evaluating environmental factors in making school siting decisions. The guidelines take into account: (1) the special vulnerabilities of children to hazardous substances, (2) the possibility of contamination at a potential school site, (3) the modes of transportation available to students and staff, (4) the efficient use of energy at the location, and (5) the potential use of the location as an emergency shelter. The guidelines are applicable to a wide range of school-related facilities, including K-12 public and private schools, technical and vocational schools, and colleges and universities. They also address the need for meaningful public involvement, establishment of environmental criteria and review processes, and evaluation of nearby sources of air pollution. The guidelines also contain a quick reference guide with information on some major environmental issues like air pollution, radon gas, pesticides, and mold.

To improve environmental health in schools, OCHP has coordinated with the Department of Education, the Centers for Disease Control and Prevention, the Agency for Toxic Substances and Disease Registry, the Department of Agriculture, the Department of Defense, the Bureau of Indian Education, the White House Council on Environmental Quality, and a number of EPA offices to develop guidelines for states to protect the health of students and school staff by addressing environmental health issues commonly encountered on or around schools. As is the case with the school siting guidelines, the *Voluntary Guidelines for States: Development and Implementation of a School Environmental Health Program* are required under the Energy Independence and Security Act. The guidelines are not intended to replace existing school environmental health regulations, but they can be used as a resource in establishing school environmental health programs. The guidelines are applicable to a wide range of school-related facilities, including K-12 public and charter/private schools, technical and vocational schools. The guidelines contain best practices that states can use to help develop key partnerships that maximize existing resources. These best practices include assessing existing resources and infrastructure, determining capabilities, developing a plan, implementing the program, evaluating the program, and sustaining the program.

For example, in the early stages of developing an environmental health program, the guidance calls for states to identify a lead office to assess existing state laws, policies, or regulations that address healthy school environments. In the later stages, the guidance calls for states to determine whether program goals need to be revised or expanded and to conduct regular program evaluations. The guidelines address the cost savings and health benefits associated with adopting a school environmental health program and encourage states to work with school districts to implement healthy schools practices. Moreover, the guidelines include links to a variety of resources for states to address school environmental health issues, such as contaminants in drinking water, pest management, and noise reduction, as well as a model K-12 school environmental health program to help schools and school districts in planning their own environmental health programs.[88]

OCHP Has Worked with Local, Tribal, and Public Service Partners to Improve Children's Environmental Health in Underserved Communities

OCHP has worked with tribal, local, and public service partners to address children's environmental health issues particularly in underserved communities. For example, OCHP has, in coordination with EPA program offices, worked with the Navajo Nation to improve water quality in tribal communities, and with the American Lung Association to reduce children's exposure to air pollutants among the Oglala Sioux Tribe in South Dakota. OCHP has also worked with numerous community organizations including the Boys and Girls Clubs of America to incorporate children's health protection into community-based, after-school programs. Additionally, OCHP has awarded grants to organizations, such as the National 4-H Society, the National Family Career and Community Association, the United National Indian Tribal Youth Organization, and the Girl Scouts of the United States of America.

[88]OCHP indicated that they awarded five grants to states totaling $750,000 in the fall of 2012 for implementing state school health programs.

Additionally, OCHP has financially supported a number of children's health efforts in underserved communities across the country. According to EPA officials, OCHP awarded approximately $1.2 million in fiscal year 2011 to various entities to help them build their capacity to address children's environmental health issues in their communities. For example, the Baltimore City Health Department received a $100,000 grant for its Healthy Environments for City Kids Program, which focuses on increasing the long-term ability of Baltimore's at-risk, low-income communities to recognize and reduce children's exposures to environmental dangers, such as lead, mold, pest, carbon monoxide, and tobacco smoke. Likewise, the National Nursing Centers Consortium, in Washington, D.C., received a $100,000 grant for its prenatal and Early Childhood Provider Training Initiative. The consortium is a national organization with a mission to advance nurse-led health care through policy, consultation, programs, and applied research. The consortium used the grant to build the capacity of Washington, D.C.'s social service providers to help them ensure that low-income pregnant women and low-income families are educated about the impacts of home-based environmental health hazards and asthma triggers for children. Farm Worker Justice, a nonprofit organization that seeks to empower migrant and seasonal farm workers by, among other things, improving their living and working conditions, also received a grant award of $100,000 for its Healthy Kids, Healthy Fields project. The project involves three community-based farm worker organizations located in California, Arizona, and Florida. The grant was used to provide outreach and educational activities for families of farm workers to improve the environmental health of their children and to build the capacity of the partner organization to support future outreach to connect more farmers with local resources.

OCHP Has Worked with Medical Experts to Enhance Health Care Providers' Knowledge about Environmental Risks to Children

OCHP, in conjunction with CDC's Agency for Toxic Substances and Disease Registry, has worked with Pediatric Environmental Health Specialty Units (PEHSU) to improve health care providers' knowledge of prenatal and childhood environmental exposures. According to the PEHSU website, a PEHSU is special unit, normally based in university medical centers, aimed at improving the environmental health of children through use of a network of experts in environmental health. PEHSUs are located across the United States, Canada, and Mexico and are able to respond to requests for information and offer advice on prevention, diagnosis, management, and treatment of environmentally related health effects in children. PEHSUs include medical experts in fields, such as allergy/immunology, neurodevelopment, toxicology, and environmental medicine. They primarily provide the following services:

(1) education/community outreach on pediatric environmental health to clinicians/health professionals, clinical trainees and the general public; (2) consultation for clinicians/health professionals regarding children's environmental health concerns; and (3) referrals to appropriate resources for children with environmental health needs (see fig. 5). For example, according an OCHP official, PEHSUs used information from OCHP to help train 15,000 health care providers across the country about prenatal and childhood environmental exposures and their health implications. PEHSUs also work with federal, state, and local agencies to address children's environmental health issues in homes, schools, and communities.

Figure 5: Services Provided by Pediatric Environmental Health Specialty Units

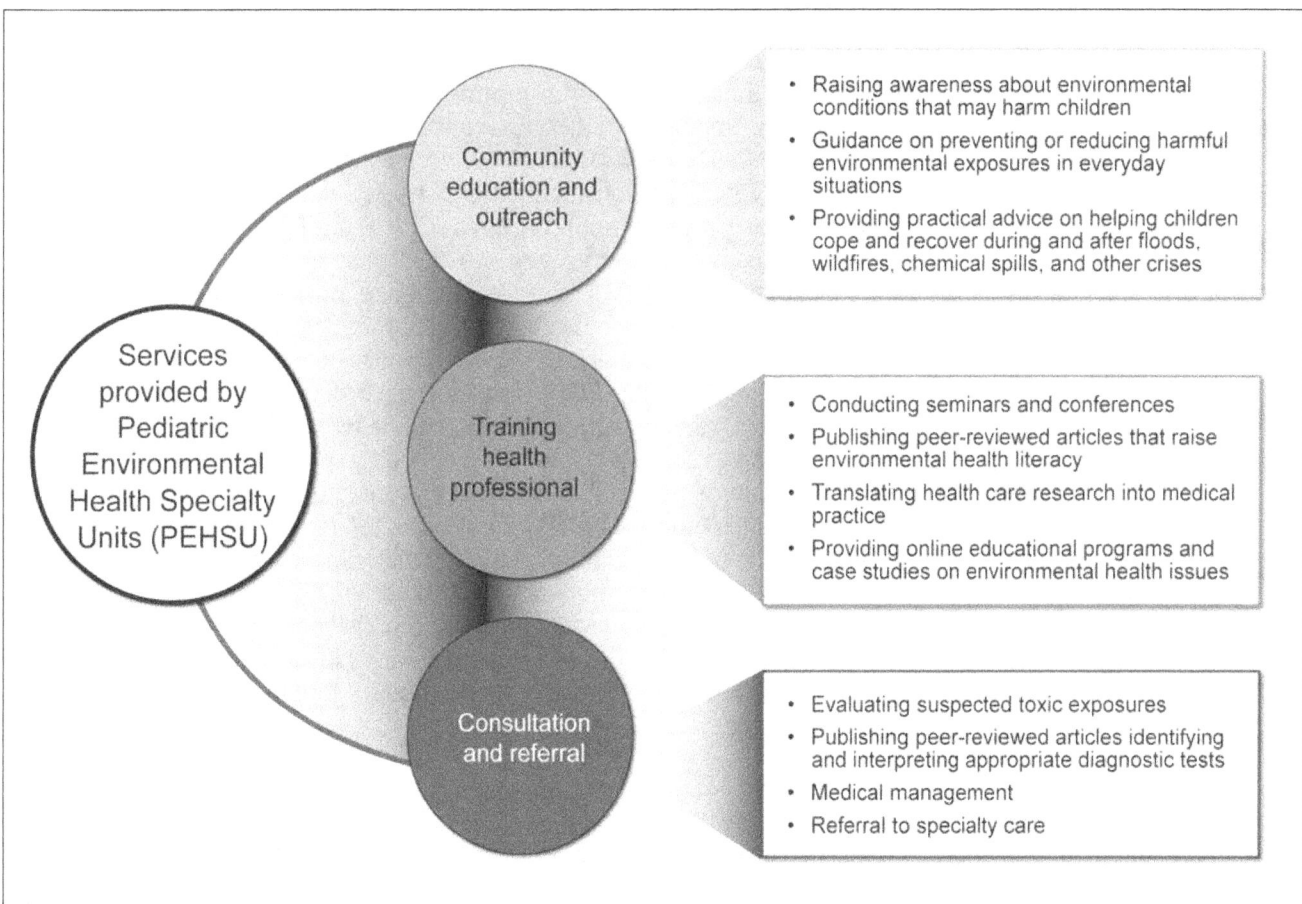

Source: GAO analysis of EPA data.

Conclusions

Protecting the health of children from environmental hazards is an integral part of EPA's mission to protect human health and the environment. EPA created OCHP to support its efforts to ensure that the agency consistently and explicitly considers children in its health protection efforts. Over the past 5 years, we have reported on numerous weaknesses in EPA's efforts to protect children's health and the many challenges the agency faces in integrating children's health protection in EPA's decision-making processes. Since our January 2010 report, EPA has made substantial progress in addressing most of our recommendations but has not fully implemented some of them. For example, EPA developed an agency-wide strategic plan that emphasizes children's health and contains a cross-cutting strategy with children-specific goals, objectives, and targets in response to our recommendations.

EPA continues, however, to struggle with several fundamental problems that we have identified in the past that may undermine the agency's ability to ensure that children's health protection is considered in all agency processes. Specifically, EPA has not taken the steps necessary to improve OCHP's ability to use the rulemaking system efficiently to identify actions potentially involving children's health, such as which regulatory workgroups would be appropriate for OCHP staff participation. EPA developed several children's health-related screening questions and included them in the ADP Tracker database, but EPA's own analysis shows that EPA rule writers are not always answering the questions consistently or accurately. EPA offers training on how to consider children's health in the ADP. However, according to Office of Policy officials, this training is not required for rule writers to understand how to respond to the screening questions related to children's health. Because of the problems associated with the screening questions in ADP Tracker, OCHP staff is manually reviewing reports to identify regulations potentially affecting children's health. Until rule writers are able to consistently and accurately answer the screening questions in ADP Tracker to identify regulatory actions potentially affecting children's health, OCHP will not be able to effectively use its resources to provide input to EPA workgroups addressing matters that may be appropriate for OCHP staff participation.

Moreover, EPA does not have a specific process for program offices that lead regulatory workgroups to document how the agency considers children's health risks in rulemakings and other actions or how their analyses comply with the 1995 Policy on Evaluating Health Risks to Children. EPA officials stated that such documentation could occur either at the preliminary analytical blueprint stage or the final agency review stage of the ADP. Without such documentation, EPA will continue to be hampered in both tracking how its regulatory actions address potential children's health issues and ensuring that the child-specific risk assessments required by the 1995 policy are being conducted.

In our January 2010 report, we recommended that EPA reevaluate its 1995 policy to ensure its consistency with the latest scientific research demonstrating the risks childhood exposures can pose for disease in later life stages. OCHP officials told us that they had reevaluated the policy and determined that it was sufficient and said that the intent of the 1995 policy was to include the best available science in the development of agency actions. EPA officials also stated that other relevant guidance documents have been updated since 1995 to ensure that current science is used to achieve the general policy and that an updated policy is not needed. However, we found that certain regulatory actions did not develop child-specific risk assessments or document why they were not done, as directed by the 1995 policy, and recommended in our May 2011 report on EPA's implementation of SDWA requirements. Rather than updating the policy, OCHP officials acknowledged that a reaffirmation of this policy could clarify that the intent of the 1995 policy was to utilize the best available science, elevate the importance of using the latest applicable guidance, and reiterate EPA's commitment to protecting children's health in the rulemaking process.

Notwithstanding the Administrator's February 2010 memorandum, which directs OCHP take the lead in ensuring that EPA program and regional offices are successful in their children's health efforts, OCHP plays no role in OPP decisions related to pesticide tolerances that can have an impact on children's health. Instead, with respect to these decisions, OPP operates independently of EPA's standard regulatory process—the ADP— and, therefore, OCHP and other program offices are not involved. OCHP officials acknowledged that, in addition to not being directly involved in pesticide decisions, they do not track, and OPP does not identify for OCHP, pesticide tolerance decisions with children's health implications. Furthermore, since OCHP has no involvement in pesticide decisions, it is not informed about changes OPP makes to margins of safety for pesticide chemical residue. Our review found that, in a large majority of cases, OPP does not use the default 10-fold safety factor for protecting children but, as allowed under FQPA, reduces the additional safety factor margins specifically established for infants and children under FQPA. While these decisions are explained by OPP in *Federal Register* notices, and assessing these decisions was outside the scope of our review, experts we spoke with have raised questions concerning the clarity of the justification provided by OPP for these decisions, while a court found EPA did not provide the requisite explanation in one instance. Experts noted as well that because the justification for these decisions may rely on CBI, a full public explanation for OPP's decision may not be possible, and one expert noted that these issues highlight the importance of having an EPA office independent of OPP—like OCHP—involved in this process. With no formal role in the pesticide tolerance decision process and no procedures to alert OCHP when matters that could pose a significant risk to children's health are being considered, it is not clear how OCHP can fully carry out its responsibilities as directed in the Administrator's February 2010 memorandum. OCHP officials acknowledged that due to limited familiarity with OPP's internal tolerance setting process and to limited staff resources they are unable to be involved in OPP actions on a regular basis, and OPP officials expressed concern regarding the practicality of involving OCHP in its pesticide tolerance decision process. Nonetheless, until the conflict between the expectations identified for OCHP in the Administrator's memorandum and the current process is addressed, OCHP's responsibilities regarding protecting children's health in the area of pesticide tolerance decisions will remain unclear.

Recommendations for Executive Action

We are recommending that the EPA Administrator take the following four actions:

- Make children's health training that includes how to respond to the screening questions a priority for rule writers.

- Require lead program offices to document their decisions in rulemakings and other actions regarding how health risks to children were considered (e.g., conducting a children's risk assessment) and that their decisions are consistent with EPA's children's health policy.

- Reaffirm the 1995 Policy on Evaluating Health Risks to Children to clarify the intent of the policy to reflect the best available science, emphasize the importance of using applicable guidance, and reiterate EPA's commitment to protecting children's health.

- Direct OCHP and OPP to establish procedures to identify tolerance decisions that could pose a significant risk to children's health and provide opportunities for OCHP involvement consistent with the Administrator's 2010 memorandum.

Agency Comments and Our Evaluation

We provided a draft of this report to EPA for its review and comment. In written comments, OCHP's Acting Director, responding on behalf of EPA, wrote that EPA generally agreed with our findings, conclusions, and recommendations. EPA's written comments on our draft report are included in appendix VI. However, EPA's comments state that the agency believes that some aspects of the report mischaracterize and underemphasize important strides that have been taken to protect children, and as a result, provided technical comments, which we incorporated into the report as appropriate.

In response to our recommendation that the EPA Administrator make children's health training that includes how to respond to the screening questions a priority for rule writers, in its comments, EPA stated that the agency is committed to exploring ways to educate rule writers. In response to our recommendation that the EPA Administrator require lead program offices to document their decisions in rulemakings and other actions regarding how health risks to children were considered (e.g., conducting a children's risk assessment) and that their decisions are consistent with EPA's children's health policy, EPA stated that OCHP works with the Office of Policy and the program offices to assure a consistent approach for documenting these decisions as part of the ADP. In response to our recommendation that the EPA Administrator reaffirm the 1995 Policy on Evaluating Health Risks to Children to clarify the intent of the policy to reflect the best available science, emphasize the importance of using applicable guidance, and reiterate EPA's commitment to protecting children's health, EPA stated that it concurred. In response to our recommendation that the EPA Administrator direct OCHP and OPP to establish procedures to identify tolerance decisions that could pose a significant risk to children's health and provide opportunities for OCHP involvement consistent with the Administrator's 2010 memorandum, EPA acknowledged the need for continued coordination and improved communication between OCHP and OPP. EPA noted that although OCHP does not participate in each tolerance decision, OPP continues to employ the framework set up to ensure that decisions appropriately consider children's health. EPA also stated that OCHP and OPP plan to develop ways to improve coordination, information sharing, prioritization, and communication and to document the agreement that is reached, thereby ensuring continued and consistent implementation. While we are encouraged by this plan, we continue to believe, as stated in our report, that until OPP and OCHP establish procedures for collaborating, OCHP's responsibilities regarding protecting children's health in the area of pesticide tolerance decisions will remain unclear.

As agreed with your office, unless you publicly announce the contents of this report earlier, we plan no further distribution until 30 days from the report date. At that time, we will send copies to the Administrator of the Environmental Protection Agency, appropriate congressional committees, and other interested parties. In addition, the report will be available at no charge on the GAO website at http://www.gao.gov.

If you or your staff members have any questions about this report, please contact me at (202) 512-3841or trimbled@gao.gov. Contact points for our Offices of Congressional Relations and Public Affairs may be found on the last page of this report. GAO staff who made major contributions to this report are listed in appendix VII.

Sincerely yours,

David C. Trimble
Director, Natural Resources and the Environment

Appendix I: Objectives, Scope, and Methodology

Our objectives were to determine (1) the extent to which the Environmental Protection Agency (EPA) has implemented our 2010 recommendations concerning children's health protection and (2) the role, if any, that the Office of Children's Health Protection (OCHP) has played in ensuring that key EPA program offices consider children's health protection in their regulatory activities. We also describe how OCHP has worked with external partners to leverage its resources to better protect children's health.

To address our first objective, we reviewed and analyzed numerous EPA documents, including the EPA Administrator's February 4, 2010, memorandum, EPA's fiscal years 2011 to 2015 strategic plan, EPA's 1995 Children Health Protection policy, OCHP's fiscal years 2011 to 2013 strategic plan, EPA's Cross-Cutting Fundamental Strategy: *Working for Environmental Justice and Children's Health*, agency action plans, and OCHP progress reports. We also compiled and analyzed official correspondence between the EPA Administrator and the Children's Health Protection Advisory Committee (CHPAC) on various children's health protection issues. Moreover, we identified key elements of several EPA databases, including ADP Tracker and RAPIDS, to determine the extent that these databases contain information that addressed our recommendations. We interviewed officials from OCHP, Office of Policy, and regional offices concerning the status of GAO's 2010 recommendations on children's health protection. We also spoke with the Co-Chairs of CHPAC to obtain their views on these recommendations. Finally, we attended several CHPAC conferences held in November 2011 and March 2012, respectively, to observe EPA involvement in CHPAC.

To address our second objective, and to better understand OCHP's role and responsibilities in EPA's Action Development Process (ADP), which the agency uses to develop rules, regulations, and other agency actions, we relied on OCHP's analysis from fiscal year 2011 based on the measures included in its fiscal years 2011 to 2013 strategic plan. As of September 2011, there were 106 regulations listed in EPA's publicly available regulatory tracking system, Reg DAART, 31 of which had not been completed and were marked by the lead program office as having a potential impact on children's health. OCHP measured its office's impact in ADP by determining whether an action that had been identified as having a potential impact on children's health was "fully responsive" to Executive Order 13045 and EPA's Children's Health Policy in addressing children's vulnerabilities. We chose to more closely examine 6 of the 31 regulations that were completed shortly after the end of fiscal year 2011 and were representative of a range of outcomes—from OCHP serving on

a workgroup for which the action was fully responsive to OCHP not
serving on a workgroup for which the action was not fully responsive. For
the 6 regulations we examined more closely, we interviewed the OCHP
representative, when there was one, and the workgroup Chair from the
lead program office, to understand the dynamics of the workgroup and
the contribution that OCHP may have made to the development of these
actions. In addition, we interviewed officials from OCHP, as well as from
several program offices that serve as the lead on actions, which could
have a potential impact on children's health. These program offices
included the Offices of Air, Water, Chemical Safety and Pollution
Prevention, and Solid Waste and Emergency Response. We also
interviewed officials from the Office of Policy, which is a core office in the
ADP, according to EPA guidance. In addition to our general discussion
about OCHP's role in the ADP, we examined OCHP's role in EPA's
implementation of two statutory requirements that explicitly require
special consideration of children—the Safe Drinking Water Act (SDWA)
and the Food Quality Protection Act (FQPA). We interviewed officials
from the lead program offices in charge of following these statutes, the
Office of Water and the Office of Pesticide Programs in the Office of
Chemical Safety and Pollution Prevention. We discussed the extent to
which these offices coordinate and communicate with OCHP in their
decision-making processes, and the officials from these offices provided
documentation, when available, to demonstrate the extent to which they
consider children's health in their decision making processes. We also
interviewed OCHP officials to better understand the level of
communication and collaboration between them and officials from the
Office of Water and the Office of Pesticide Programs. To gain an outside
perspective on the highly technical issue of how the Office of Pesticide
Programs' pesticide registration and tolerance decisions meet FQPA
criteria to consider children's exposure, we selected a nonprobability
sample of eight academic, medical, and industry experts in the field of
children's environmental health, pesticide exposure, and implementation
of FQPA to interview. We selected these eight experts based on several
factors including their current representation on EPA's CHPAC or EPA's
Pesticide Program Dialogue Committee (PPDC). The Office of Pesticide
Programs (OPP) provided us with summary information from its ISTEP
MS Access database that tracks the most recent FQPA safety factor
applied in an EPA risk assessment from 1996—the year that FQPA was
enacted—to 2012. We assessed the reliability of the summary data on
these decisions by (1) reviewing existing information about the data and
the system that produced them and (2) interviewing agency officials
knowledgeable about the data. We determined that the data were
sufficiently reliable for the purposes of this report.

To address our third objective, we reviewed various EPA documents related to children's health protection, including EPA's healthy homes strategy, *Advancing Healthy Housing: A Strategy for Action*, and key voluntary guidance issued by EPA for schools: *School Siting Guidelines and Voluntary Guidelines for States: Development and Implementation of a School Environmental Health Program*. We also reviewed a draft presentation of the healthy homes website, scheduled to be launched in 2013 by the Department of Housing and Urban Development, as well as information from the Association of Occupational and Environmental Clinics' website on Pediatric Environmental Health Specialty Units and the role these units play in helping to improve the knowledge of health care providers on prenatal and childhood environmental exposures. Moreover, we reviewed OCHP grant data from fiscal years 2011 and 2012 associated with activities in support of children's health protection, as well as OCHP progress reports highlighting the office's accomplishments relative to activities outline in its strategic plan. We interviewed officials from OCHP, particularly officials within OCHP's Program Implementation and Coordination Division and EPA's Office of Budget about the external activities that support children's health protections, as well as the resources dedicated to children's health-related outreach and coordination. We interviewed representatives from several nongovernmental organizations, including representatives from the National Center for Health Housing, the Natural Resources Defense Council, the Health and Environment Program National Environmental Education Foundation, the Healthy Schools Network, Incorporated, and the 21 Century School Fund and Building Educational Success Together to obtain their views on the effectiveness of OCHP's outreach and coordination efforts pertaining to children's health.

We conducted this performance audit from November 2011 to August 2013 in accordance with generally accepted government auditing standards. Those standards require that we plan and perform the audit to obtain sufficient, appropriate evidence to provide a reasonable basis for our findings and conclusions based on our audit objectives. We believe that the evidence obtained provides a reasonable basis for our findings and conclusions based on our audit objectives.

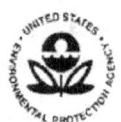

UNITED STATES ENVIRONMENTAL PROTECTION AGENCY
WASHINGTON, D.C. 20460

OFFICE OF
THE ADMINISTRATOR

OCT 20 1995

MEMORANDUM

SUBJECT: New Policy on Evaluating Health Risks to Children

TO: Assistant Administrators
        General Counsel
        Inspector General
        Associate Administrators
        Regional Administrators

We are establishing a new Agency-wide policy (attached) that will, for the first time, ensure that we consistently and explicitly evaluate environmental health risks of infants and children in all of the risk assessments, risk characterizations, and environmental and public health standards that we set for the nation.

This is not a new idea to the many programs throughout the Agency that currently consider children's health issues in assessing overall risk. This is, however, a major step forward in establishing a consistent nationwide children's environmental health policy. We know that children have a greater potential for exposure to environmental hazards and our assessments of health risks do not always fully take into account the potential effects on this vulnerable population. The National Academy of Sciences has called for policy changes to reflect children's health factors in evaluating environmental risks.

Our new policy answers that call for change and, in doing so, will allow us to make better public health decisions that reflect not just data on adults, but on children whenever possible. By making children a health priority, we expect that this policy will encourage new, much-needed research to provide the child-specific data we will need to thoroughly evaluate the health risks children and infants face from pollution in our air, land, and water. In the long run, healthier children mean healthier adults - a great benefit for the nation.

The policy set forth in this memorandum takes effect November 1, 1995, and is sponsored by the Agency's Science Policy Council, which is charged with evaluating science policy issues of Agency-wide importance. We are confident that each of your offices will work with the Council to ensure a smooth transition to this new policy that is so important to our nation's future.

/s/   /s/
Carol M. Browner   Fred Hansen
Administrator   Deputy Administrator

Attachment

Policy on Evaluating
Health Risks to Children

POLICY

It is the policy[1] of the U.S. Environmental Protection Agency (EPA) to consider the risks to infants and children consistently and explicitly as a part of risk assessments generated during its decision making process, including the setting of standards to protect public health and the environment. To the degree permitted by available data in each case, the Agency will develop a separate assessment of risks to infants and children or state clearly why this is not done - for example, a demonstration that infants and children are not expected to be exposed to the stressor under examination.

BACKGROUND

When it comes to their health and development, children are not little adults. This maxim has long been understood in the medical community. Documentation of the similarities and differences between children and adults is an integral part of assessing the effects and efficacy of drugs, for example. The National Academy of Sciences has pointed out on more than one occasion[2,3] that the maxim should hold true with respect to exposure to environmental pollutants, as well.

Children may be more or less sensitive than adults when confronted with an equivalent level of exposure to an environmental pollutant. In many cases, their responses are substantially different - qualitatively and quantitatively - from those exhibited by adults. These age-related variations in susceptibility are due to many factors, including differences in pharmacokinetics, pharmacodynamics, body composition, and maturity of biochemical and physiological functions (for example, metabolic rates and pathways).

In addition, there are often age-related differences in types and levels of exposure. For example, it is known that infants and children differ from adults both qualitatively and quantitatively in their exposures to pesticides in foods. Children eat more food and drink more water per unit of body weight, and the variety of the food they consume is more limited than adults. Children also breathe more rapidly than adults and can inhale more of an air pollutant per pound of body weight than adults. Children's skin and other body tissues may absorb some harmful substances more easily. Children's bodies are not yet fully developed, so exposure to toxic substances may affect their growth and development. Infants' immune systems are not as strong as those of healthy adults, so they are less able to fight off emerging microbial threats such as Cryptosporidium in drinking water.

The Agency is particularly concerned about safeguarding the health of infants and children, who are among the nation's most fragile and vulnerable populations. Therefore, it is important that there be a clear articulation of policy in this regard.

IMPLEMENTATION

---

[1] This document is a statement of Agency policy and does not constitute a rule. It is not intended, nor can it be relied upon, to create any rights enforceable by any party in litigation with the United States.

[2] National Research Council. 1993. Pesticides in the Diets of Infants and Children. National Academy of Sciences Press, Washington, DC.

[3] National Research Council. 1994. Science and Judgment in Risk Assessment. National Academy of Sciences Press, Washington, DC.

The policy already is currently being followed in many Programs and regions. The entire Agency will expand implementation activities during the Fall of 1995 as part of the overall implementation of the Administrator's policy on risk characterization. Other related activities and sources of information include the presentation of relevant data in the revised draft Exposure Factors Handbook, and current EPA solicitations of grant proposals for independent studies on risk to children from exposure to a wide range of substances. EPA's 1991 Guidelines for Developmental Toxicity Risk Assessment are also relevant.

This policy is not retroactive; it will apply only to those assessments started or revised on or after November 1, 1995. Any questions relating to the policy and its implementation should be referred to Dr. Dorothy Patton, Executive Director of the Agency's Science Policy Council. She can be reached at 202-260-6600.

Appendix III: EPA Administrator's February 2010 Memorandum

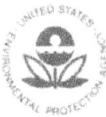

UNITED STATES ENVIRONMENTAL PROTECTION AGENCY
WASHINGTON, D.C. 20460

FEB 4 2010

THE ADMINISTRATOR

MEMORANDUM

SUBJECT: EPA's Leadership in Children's Environmental Health

FROM: Lisa P. Jackson
Administrator

TO: Assistant Administrators
Associate Administrators
General Counsel
Regional Administrators

Protecting children's environmental health is central to our work at EPA. As we move ahead on critical environmental initiatives and sharpen our focus on our seven priorities for EPA's future, we must ensure that children's health protection is a driving force in our decisions.

Let me reaffirm that it is EPA's policy to consider the health of pregnant women, infants and children consistently and explicitly in all activities we undertake related to human-health protection, both domestically and internationally. This includes consistently following Agency policies to account for specific exposure pathways and dose-response characteristics of children in our risk assessments and standard setting practices.

Research has demonstrated that prenatal and early-life exposures to environmental contaminants can have tragic, life-long effects. Children's neurological, immunological, digestive, and other bodily systems are still developing; children eat more food, drink more fluids, and breathe more air in proportion to their body weight than adults; and children's behavior patterns can make them more susceptible to environmental exposures. We must be diligent in our efforts to ensure that dangerous exposures and health risks to children are prevented.

EPA will use a variety of approaches to protect children from environmental health hazards. Those approaches will include regulation, implementation of community-based programs, research, and outreach. At the same time, we must periodically evaluate our performance to ensure that we are making steady progress.

The Office of Children's Health Protection in the Administrator's Office will take the lead in ensuring that the programs and Regions are successful in their efforts to protect children's health. Please contact Office Director, Peter Grevatt if you need assistance in your efforts to make children's environmental health a priority in all Agency programs and actions.

EPA's Children's Health Agenda

EPA's children's health-protection efforts are guided by Executive Order 13045 (Protection of Children from Environmental Health Risks and Safety Risks), its Policy on Evaluating Health Risks to Children (1995), the *Guide to Considering Children's Health When Developing Agency Actions,* various statutory requirements, and the best available research and data on children's health risks.

Following are three key areas in EPA's agenda to both focus and ensure that the Agency's actions address the environmental origins of health problems in children and are protective of children's environmental health:

First, our efforts to implement the nation's environmental laws must use the best science to include a focus on children. We will robustly and transparently address the potential for and uniqueness of health effects in children during the development of regulations and Agency policies with human-health implications. We will work with states and tribes to ensure that regulations are effectively implemented and enforced to protect children's health. We will also work closely with external research partners to fill critical data gaps on children's.

Second, we will protect children through safe chemicals management. I named chemical management as one of our top priorities for EPA's future largely because of the disproportionate effects of chemical exposures on children. We will establish standards, policies and guidance at home and abroad that help eliminate harmful prenatal and childhood exposures to pesticides and other toxic chemicals. We will work with Congress and stakeholders to identify effective approaches for the protection of children's health in the context of TSCA reform. We will also encourage green chemistry and safer alternatives to chemicals and products that present a potential hazard to children.

Third, we will coordinate national and international community-based programs to eliminate threats to children's health and measure and communicate progress. We will expand implementation of successful community-based programs to protect and improve children's health outcomes. That effort will focus on underserved communities, including tribes and other areas where children's health is at heightened risk. The Office of Children's Health Protection will work with program offices and regions to develop and track indicators of progress in protecting children's health, and we will communicate that progress to the public.

I look forward to working with you to ensure that children's health is paramount at EPA.

cc: Bob Perciasepe
Diane Thompson
Bob Sussman
Ray Spears
Lisa Garcia
Larry Elworth
Peter Grevatt

Appendix IV: Office of Children's Health Protection's Involvement in Agency Actions in Fiscal Year 2011

Table 1 depicts ongoing EPA actions in fiscal year 2011 that program offices identified as having a potential impact on children's health. During this time period OCHP was involved in 21 of the 31 workgroups addressing these actions. There were four program offices that had the lead role in the development of these EPA actions, as depicted below.

Table 1: Agency Actions Addressing Children's Health in Fiscal Year 2011

Agency action	OCHP on workgroup?	Lead program office
Control of Air Pollution From Motor Vehicles: Tier 3 Motor Vehicle Emission and Fuel Standards	Yes	OAR
Formaldehyde Emissions Standards for Composite Wood Products	Yes	OCSPP
Lead Emissions from Piston-Engine Aircraft Using Leaded Aviation Gasoline	Yes	OAR
Lead Wheel Weights; Regulatory Investigation	Yes	OCSPP
*Lead; Clearance and Clearance Testing Requirements for the Renovation, Repair, and Painting Program (completed 8/11)	Yes	OCSPP
Lead; Renovation, Repair, and Painting Program for Public and Commercial Buildings	Yes	OCSPP
Lead; Residential Lead Dust Hazard Standards	Yes	OCSPP
Long-Chain Perfluorinated Chemicals (LCPFCs); Regulation(s) Under TSCA	Yes	OCSPP
National Primary Drinking Water Regulations for Lead and Copper: Regulatory Revisions	Yes	OW
National Primary Drinking Water Regulations: Regulation of Perchlorate	Yes	OW
Pesticides; Agricultural Worker Protection Standard Revisions	Yes	OCSPP
Pesticides; Certification of Pesticide Applicators	Yes	OCSPP
*Review of the National Ambient Air Quality Standards for Carbon Monoxide (completed 8/11)	Yes	OAR
Review of the National Ambient Air Quality Standards for Lead	Yes	OAR
Review of the National Ambient Air Quality Standards for Ozone	Yes	OAR
Review of the National Ambient Qir Quality Standards for Particulate Matter	Yes	OAR
*Revision to Pb Ambient Air Monitoring Requirements (completed 12/10)	Yes	OAR
Revisions to EPA's Rule on Protections for Subjects in Human Research Involving Pesticides	Yes	OCSPP
*Control of Greenhouse Gas Emissions from Medium and Heavy-Duty Vehicles (completed 9/11)	Yes	OAR
Joint Rulemaking to Establish 2017 and Later Model Year Light Duty Vehicle GHG Emissions and CAFÉ Standards	Yes	OAR
Reconsideration of the 2008 Ozone Primary and Secondary National Ambient Air Quality Standards	Yes	OAR
Mercury; Regulation of Use in Certain Products	No	OCSPP
*NESHAP for Primary Lead Smelting (completed 11/11)	No	OAR
Addition of Vapor Intrusion Component to the Hazard Ranking System (HRS)	No	OSWER

Appendix IV: Office of Children's Health
Protection's Involvement in Agency Actions in
Fiscal Year 2011

Agency action	OCHP on workgroup?	Lead program office
NESHAP: Mercury Cell Chlor-Alkali Plants - Amendments	No	OAR
Remand of Halogenated Solvent Cleaning Final Residual Risk Rule	No	OAR
*Residual Risk and Technology Review for Secondary Lead Smelters NESHAP (completed 1/12)	No	OAR
Risk and Technology Review for Ferroalloys Production	No	OAR
Risk and Technology Review for National Emission Standards for Hazardous Air Pollutants from the Pulp and Paper Industry	No	OAR
Rulemaking on the Definition of Solid Waste	No	OSWER
Standards for the Management of Coal Combustion Residuals Generated by Commercial Electric Power Producers	No	OSWER

Source: EPA Office of Children's Health Protection.

The * designates agency actions that were finalized shortly after fiscal year 2011 during the time period of GAO's review. GAO examined these actions more closely by interviewing workgroup chairs from the lead program offices and relevant OCHP program representatives. We refer to these actions in the body of the report.

Note: The acronyms in the above table represent the following EPA program offices: OAR, Office of Air and Radiation; OSCPP, Office of Chemical Safety and Pollution Prevention; OW, Office of Water; and OSWER, Office of Solid Waste and Emergency Response.

Appendix V: FQPA Tolerance Decisions by OPP for Fiscal Year 2011

OPP officials provided us with the rationale associated with tolerance decisions for one year— fiscal year 2011. OPP provided a summary table listing each tolerance decision, the FQPA safety factor applied, and a phrase indicating the rationale only for those tolerance decisions where OPP retained all (default 10-fold) or part (3-fold) of the FQPA safety factor.[1] The fiscal year 2011 data indicated all the FQPA safety factor decisions to retain all or part of the safety factor were made based on one of the following three rationales:

(1) the use of a "lowest observed adverse effect level (LOAEL)" instead of a "no observed adverse effect level;"[2] for the three 3-fold safety factor decisions in fiscal year 2011, this was the reason cited;

(2) a data gap, meaning one or more required toxicity study was not complete, such as an inhalation study or developmental toxicity study; and

(3) studies did not test the required duration of exposure, and extrapolation was required.

In fiscal year 2011 all but 9 of the 57 tolerance decisions applied a 1-fold safety factor. For 3 of the 9 decisions, a 3-fold safety factor was applied, and all of them were due to the use of a LOAEL. For the remaining 6 decisions, all 4 applied a 10-fold safety factor. Of the 6 10-fold safety factor decisions, 1 was due to a LOAEL, 4 were due to a data gap, and 1 was due to studies that did not test the required duration of exposure.

---

[1]OPP officials did not provide similar rationale for every 1-fold decision from fiscal year 2011 in the written documentation provided to GAO.

[2]According to EPA, lowest observed adverse effect level is the lowest dose in a toxicity study resulting in adverse health effects. Conversely, no observed adverse effect level is the highest dose in a toxicity study that does not result in adverse health effects and thus does not cause observable harm.

Appendix VI: Comments from the Environmental Protection Agency

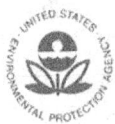

UNITED STATES ENVIRONMENTAL PROTECTION AGENCY
WASHINGTON, D.C. 20460

JUN 2 1 2013

OFFICE OF
CHILDREN'S HEALTH PROTECTION

Mr. Alfredo Gomez
Director
Natural Resources and Environment
U.S. Government Accountability Office
Washington, DC 20548

Dear Mr. Gomez:

Thank you for the opportunity to review and comment on the Government Accountability Office (GAO) draft report, entitled: *EPA Has Made Substantial Progress but Could Improve Processes for Considering Children's Health* (GAO-13-254). The purpose of this letter is to provide the Environmental Protection Agency (EPA, agency) response to your recommendations and to provide technical comments (attached). The EPA generally agrees with the GAO's recommendations.

Since its inception, EPA has made protecting children's environmental health part of our mission. As the draft report highlights, the agency has made substantial progress in its effort to consider children's health. Since the 2010 GAO report, the Office of Children's Health Protection (OCHP) was reorganized to increase the agency's focus on children's health. Prior to the reorganization, OCHP's mission was broader and included a focus on both aging and environmental education. Also, in February 2010, the Administrator issued a memorandum that reaffirmed the agency's commitment to children's health.

As recommended by GAO, the agency-wide strategic plan for fiscal years 2011–2015 identifies children's health as a top priority. In addition, the agency more specifically discusses how it plans to address children's health in the Cross-Cutting Fundamental Strategy: Working for Environmental Justice and Children's Health. Each year an action plan is developed that lists specific tasks that will be taken in carrying out the principles of the cross-cutting strategy. OCHP also finalized an office strategic plan for fiscal years 2011-2013. The plan defines a vision and mission for the office, establishes goals and objectives for their implementation, and describes measures for evaluating progress.

GAO correctly points out that OCHP has also strengthened its relationships with external partners. OCHP proactively uses the Children's Health Protection Advisory Committee

Internet Address (URL) • http://www.epa.gov
Recycled/Recyclable • Printed with Vegetable Oil Based Inks on 100% Postconsumer, Process Chlorine Free Recycled Paper

(CHPAC) to provide advice on regulations, policies and other issues. For example, the CHPAC recently sent a letter to the Administrator that provided advice on childhood lead poisoning prevention programs. Furthermore, OCHP has actively participated in the interagency organizations initiated under Executive Order 13045 (the President's Task Force on Environmental Health Risks and Safety Risks to Children (Task Force) and the Federal Interagency Forum on Child and Family Statistics (Forum)). The Task Force released the *Coordinated Federal Action Plan to Reduce Racial and Ethnic Asthma Disparities* after coordination with the CHPAC, many federal agencies and external partners. The Task Force also made significant contributions regarding children's health to *Advancing Healthy Housing – A Strategy for Action* released by the federal Healthy Homes Work Group (OCHP is a member of this group). Finally, EPA has consistently participated in the Forum. The Forum is a working group of federal agencies that collect, analyze and report data on conditions and trends related to children and family well-being. The agency has contributed to several of the Forum's reports including *America's Children* (2011) and *America's Children in Brief: Key National Indicators of Well-Being* (2012) and is currently working on the 2013 edition of *America's Children.*

GAO's review of children's health in regulatory efforts at EPA focused on two statutory requirements – the Safe Drinking Water Act (SDWA) and the Food Quality Protection Act (FQPA) -- and OCHP's role in developing drinking water standards and pesticide tolerance decisions with adequate margins of safety. The report also discussed where children are considered in the Action Development Process (ADP). We agree with the report's conclusions that OCHP has played a more active role in SDWA actions but additional efforts are needed regarding FQPA actions. However, the agency has long established policies and frameworks to ensure consideration of particular vulnerabilities of children in decision-making under FQPA and for pesticide food tolerance setting.

The draft report also highlights the work OCHP has done with external partners to leverage resources to better protect children's health. Along with the previously mentioned *Advancing Healthy Housing – A Strategy for Action*, OCHP has worked with the National Center for Healthy Housing to promote training initiatives. OCHP has also worked with partners to implement several programs related to schools as required under the Energy Independence and Security Act (EISA) of 2007. OCHP released *Voluntary School Siting Guidelines* and *Voluntary Guidelines for States: Development and Implementation of a School Environmental Health Program* as well as implemented a grant program for state agencies. Through another grant program, OCHP financially supported a number of children's health efforts in underserved communities (including tribal communities) across the country. These capacity building grants funded projects that are addressing issues encountered by migrant and seasonal farm workers, low-income pregnant women and children, among others. OCHP also works with the Centers for Disease Control and Prevention's Agency for Toxic Substances and Disease Registry to support Pediatric Environmental Health Specialty Units (PEHSUs) throughout the country.

2

While EPA generally agrees with the recommendations of GAO, we believe that some aspects of the report mischaracterize and under-emphasize important strides that have been taken to protect children. Therefore we have enclosed corrections to technical inaccuracies and clarifications regarding potentially misleading statements or characterizations (see Attachment 1). In an effort to ensure that preparers and recipients of this report use consistent terminology, we have added a clarification of terms (see Attachment 2). Also as a means to provide background and reference information regarding lawsuits under FQPA and pesticide tolerances, we have enclosed a review of select legal actions under FQPA (see Attachment 3) and Amisulbrom as an example of an important tolerance (see Attachment 4).

GAO Recommendation 1: Make children's health training that includes how to respond to the screening questions a priority for rule writers.

EPA Response: The EPA is committed to exploring ways to educate rule writers. Recently OCHP worked with the Office of Policy (OP) to update the children's health segment of the *Action Development at EPA* training course. This class targets new EPA rule writers and provides guidance on methods for ensuring children's unique vulnerabilities are appropriately considered in EPA's regulatory actions. In the FY 2013 Action Plan for the agency's Cross Cutting Fundamental Strategy: Working for Environmental Justice and Children's Health, OCHP is tasked with developing an additional webinar-based training available to all EPA staff, but targeting rule developers. The purpose of this training is to enhance the understanding of how to apply children's environmental health principles within EPA's regulatory process. The training course has been developed and is currently being reviewed internally. OCHP is on course to meet the September 2013 deadline established in the strategy. Both courses cover how to respond to children's health screening questions in the ADP. OCHP believes that this combination of classes will ensure that rule writers are properly trained.

GAO Recommendation 2: Require lead program offices to document their decisions in rulemakings and other actions regarding how health risks to children were considered (e.g., conducting a children's risk assessment) and that their decisions are consistent with EPA's children's health policy.

EPA Response: EPA agrees with the importance of ensuring that decisions regarding children's health risks in rulemakings are consistent with EPA's policy on children's health and documenting those decisions. OCHP will work with OP and other program offices to assure a consistent approach for documenting these decisions as a part of the ADP at EPA.

3

GAO Recommendation 3: Reaffirm the 1995 Policy on Evaluating Health Risks to Children to clarify the intent of the policy to reflect the best available science, emphasize the importance of using applicable guidance and reiterate EPA's commitment to protecting children's health.

EPA Response: EPA concurs with the idea of reaffirming the 1995 Policy. In fact, we believe this reaffirmation could be a periodic activity; by so doing, the policy never goes out of date and is routinely highlighted as an agency priority. OCHP will work with the Acting or new Administrator to draft a memo that reaffirms the 1995 Policy and the mission of OCHP.

GAO Recommendation 4: Direct the Office of Children's Health Protection (OCHP) and the Office of Pesticide Programs (OPP) to establish procedures to identify tolerance decisions that could pose a significant risk to children's health and provide opportunities for OCHP involvement consistent with the Administrator's 2010 memorandum.

EPA Response: EPA acknowledges the need for continued coordination and improved communication between OCHP and OPP. The framework within which pesticide tolerance setting occurs was established after the passage of FQPA in 1996, and incorporated intra-agency participation and federal advisory committee consultation, including consultation with the Scientific Advisory Panel (SAP), and the Pesticide Program Dialogue Committee (PPDC). This resulted in a policy and scientific framework that was protective of children's health. Even though OCHP does not participate in each tolerance decision, OPP continues to employ the framework set up to ensure that decisions appropriately consider children's health. OCHP and OPP are committed to ensuring that the agency fully complies with the 1995 Policy and have already begun to discuss ways to improve coordination, information sharing, prioritization and communication. The two organizations plan to document the agreement that is reached, thereby ensuring continued and consistent implementation.

The EPA generally agrees with the findings, conclusions, and recommendations and thanks the GAO for the opportunity to review the draft report. Please feel free to contact Khesha Reed at (202) 566-0594 if you have questions or need further information.

Jacqueline Mosby, MPH
Acting Director
Office of Children's Health Protection

4

Attachments

cc: Vanessa Bowie, OCFO
       Patricia Gilchriest, OES
       Michael Goo, OP
       Jim Jones, OCSPP
       William Nickerson, OP
       Khesha Reed, OCHP
       Janet Wiener, OCSPP

5

Appendix VII: GAO Contact and Staff Acknowledgments

GAO Contact	David C. Trimble, (202) 512-3841 or trimbled@gao.gov
Staff Acknowledgments	In addition to the individual named above, Diane B. Raynes, Assistant Director; Elizabeth Beardsley; Mark Braza; John C. Johnson; Celia Mendive; and Amy Ward-Meier made significant contributions to this report. Cheryl Arvidson, Armetha Liles, Cynthia Norris, and Kiki Theodoropoulos also made important contributions to this report.

GAO's Mission	The Government Accountability Office, the audit, evaluation, and investigative arm of Congress, exists to support Congress in meeting its constitutional responsibilities and to help improve the performance and accountability of the federal government for the American people. GAO examines the use of public funds; evaluates federal programs and policies; and provides analyses, recommendations, and other assistance to help Congress make informed oversight, policy, and funding decisions. GAO's commitment to good government is reflected in its core values of accountability, integrity, and reliability.
Obtaining Copies of GAO Reports and Testimony	The fastest and easiest way to obtain copies of GAO documents at no cost is through GAO's website (http://www.gao.gov). Each weekday afternoon, GAO posts on its website newly released reports, testimony, and correspondence. To have GAO e-mail you a list of newly posted products, go to http://www.gao.gov and select "E-mail Updates."
Order by Phone	The price of each GAO publication reflects GAO's actual cost of production and distribution and depends on the number of pages in the publication and whether the publication is printed in color or black and white. Pricing and ordering information is posted on GAO's website, http://www.gao.gov/ordering.htm. Place orders by calling (202) 512-6000, toll free (866) 801-7077, or TDD (202) 512-2537. Orders may be paid for using American Express, Discover Card, MasterCard, Visa, check, or money order. Call for additional information.
Connect with GAO	Connect with GAO on Facebook, Flickr, Twitter, and YouTube. Subscribe to our RSS Feeds or E-mail Updates. Listen to our Podcasts. Visit GAO on the web at www.gao.gov.
To Report Fraud, Waste, and Abuse in Federal Programs	Contact: Website: http://www.gao.gov/fraudnet/fraudnet.htm E-mail: fraudnet@gao.gov Automated answering system: (800) 424-5454 or (202) 512-7470
Congressional Relations	Katherine Siggerud, Managing Director, siggerudk@gao.gov, (202) 512-4400, U.S. Government Accountability Office, 441 G Street NW, Room 7125, Washington, DC 20548
Public Affairs	Chuck Young, Managing Director, youngc1@gao.gov, (202) 512-4800 U.S. Government Accountability Office, 441 G Street NW, Room 7149 Washington, DC 20548